Feeding PICKY Kids

❧ The Natural Way to Handle Picky Eaters ❧

Christine Sullivan

B.Soc.Wk.,N.D.,D.H.M.,B.N., P.G.D.H.Sc (Nutrition Medicine)
Naturopath, Nutrition Medicine Practitioner, Herbalist & 'KIDEOLOGY' specialist

Disclaimer

The information in this book is provided for educational and informational purposes only, and is not intended to be a substitute for a health care provider's consultation. Please consult your own physician or appropriate health care provider about the applicability of any opinions or recommendations with respect to your own situation. This book should not be considered complete, nor should it be relied on to suggest a course of treatment for a particular individual. It should not be used in place of consultation or advice from a physician or other qualified health care provider.

First edition
Copyright © Christine Sullivan
Copyright photographs © individual photographer's
ISBN 978-0-9925539-0-6

This edition published by Whole Happiness Publishing
PO Box 2208, Byron Bay, NSW, Australia

CONTENTS

A PERSONAL MESSAGE

Does family mealtime feel like a battlefield?
Do you need ideas to incorporate healthy foods into your picky eater's diet?
Do you want the best nutrition possible for your child?
Of course you do! We all want the best for our children.

Thank you for choosing to buy my guide to feeding picky kids and children who won't eat. I hope that it will give you some tools and strategies to deal with your picky and fussy eaters, reduce the stress around mealtimes and help you ensure the best nutrition for your child.

Here you will find useful information, tips, tricks and tools to deal with your picky kids from the normally fussy toddler through to the older more resistant eaters.

My absolute passion is assisting parents in every way possible to ensure that their children are the healthiest and happiest they can be, to reach their true potential and live healthy fulfilling lives. Every day, I assist prospective parents to reach ideal nutrition before conceiving the healthiest possible child. I support women through their pregnancy, birth and lactation and then continue to support the parenting of their much loved children.

So many parents are concerned about their children being picky eaters. Even the most health conscious parents, no matter how hard they try, can have a hard time making sure their kids eat the right foods and get the right level of nutrition to keep them healthy.

Over the past two and a half decades I have worked with thousands of families struggling with many different aspects of raising children. Picky and fussy eating behaviour has always been a major area of concern as it can have so many implications.

In dealing with children's health I have developed a concept that I call 'KIDEOLOGY'. To me, KIDEOLOGY is the art and science of treating children holistically with good nutrition and with natural food as their medicine where ever possible. This e-book encompasses my KIDEOLOGY philosophy.

Because I have seen such wonderful outcomes working with my young picky eaters I thought that this book would be an excellent opportunity to share with you not only my experiences of being the ultimate picky eater as a child myself, but also as a parent of three beautiful (and sometimes very picky!) children as well as a naturopath and nutrition medicine consultant with more than 28 years of experience treating children and their family's health and dietary issues.

Through this book I hope to help parents everywhere deal with this issue. Working with children can be very challenging at times but at the same time it is immensely rewarding.

They can be quite fragile little beings and yet are enormously resilient and respond quickly to the right food and environment.

I will take you through the reasons that may be behind your child's picky eating, mealtime strategies to try, lots of imaginative ways to include nutrient dense foods to ensure your child gets their required nutrients, hints on educating your child about food and some nutrition fundamentals so you can choose the best foods for a happy healthy child.

Children can typically go through stages of disinterest in food and eating and this is of course very worrying for parents, as proper nutrition is essential for normal growth and development. However children's appetites can vary naturally depending on their growth needs.

Whether your child is just going through the fussy toddler stage or if their fussiness and pickiness regarding food is more entrenched, my aim here is to calm the worry that I know you will be going through.

Parent's efforts and involvement is a major factor in the successful treatment outcomes when working with children. I salute all of you out there for your persistence. You are such an important influence in your children's lives and I want to support you in your parenting role as much as I possibly can. To me, being a parent is the most important job in the world.

Feeding Picky Kids is designed for ALL parents wanting to ensure their child eats well and can be applied to all levels of picky eating and for children of all ages. Feel free to skip ahead and read the chapters of most interest to you first and then come back and read through the rest for more ideas and understanding.

I hope you will find some answers and helpful strategies here in this book.

Wishing you great success.

Chris

CHAPTER 1
WHAT IS A PICKY EATER EXACTLY

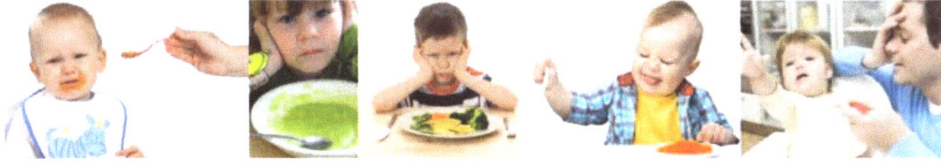

Can We Define It?

Does your child fuss and reject food once in a while or do you have daily battles at meal times? I see picky eating on a continuum with the occasional toddler or fusspot eating at one end and more difficult selective eating and food rejection at the other and many variations in between.

Occasionally fussy or picky with food ◄——► *Extremely picky & very selective with food*

Let's look at some definitions.

The term *picky eater* has been defined in a number of different ways.

In 1990 Marchi and Cohen defined picky eating by the presence of three of the following child behaviours

- *does not eat enough*
- *is often or very often choosy about food*
- *usually eats slowly*
- *is usually not interested in food*

To me, this definition covers the milder (left side) of my continuum and is very typical of toddlerhood. It covers those children who do eat most of the time but may only eat a couple of very specific meals and nothing else. For instance, won't eat any vegetable, won't eat any fruit, will not eat green things or will only eat white foods.

On the other hand, in 1997 Timimi, Douglas and Tsiftsopoulou, looking at children aged 4 to 14 years defined fussy and picky eating as:

> *"A specific and persistent pattern of behaviour consisting of a refusal to eat any foods outside of a limited range of preferred foods."*

They also included accompanying behaviours such as resisting attempts at self-feeding, gagging, spitting out food, mealtime disruptive behaviours, playing with food at mealtimes, excessively slow eating and difficulties swallowing or chewing food. This definition seems to sway toward the more severe end of the continuum.

Once, a picky eater was defined as one who would only eat a limited number of foods but, for the most part, those foods would have been real foods.

For children today the risk is that picky eating may mean that they will only eat highly processed, high energy but nutrient devoid fast foods and convenience snacks such as crisps, crackers, processed cereals and such.

So at a time when the food that your child would rather eat highly processed, additive laden and lacking the vital nutrients that a small body needs to grow and develop, it is vital that fussy or picky eating is addressed as soon as possible.

Is Picky Eating Common In Young Children?

Every child is unique with his or her own particular likes and dislikes which can sometimes change on a daily basis. Their overall appetite may also be equally unpredictable. Toddlers and pre-schoolers (and sometimes older children) commonly go through a stage of being very picky eaters.

Studies show that as many as 1 in 4 toddlers can be defined as food rejecters and refuse to eat what has been prepared for them at least half of the time. They may reject anything that is in any way different to what they are used to or that may be presented in a different way or they may have food fads, eating only very specific and limited favourite foods – their flavour of the month.

As long as these are relatively healthy choices there is little need to worry.

An Australian study, conducted by Gilmore in 2006, found a notable number of children displayed eating behaviours that caused considerable concern for their mothers. She found that 25% of 2-4 year olds frequently or always had food fads and 18% of those had frequent or constant picky eating. By comparison, just 16% of 7-9 year olds had food fads and around 7% were definitive picky eaters. Younger children also appeared to be more restricted in their food choices and frequently refused to try new foods.

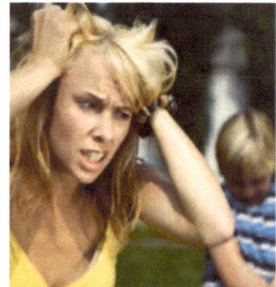

Another recent Australian study found that 82% of parents felt food rejection was a concern and that around 41% of parents are worried about their child's fussiness with food.

So, are you one of these parents?
- *Are you tearing your hair out trying to get your child to eat?*
- *Are mealtimes at your place a battle ground?*

I remember mealtimes were certainly a battle ground in my home as a child. On reflection, I was the ultimate picky eater. I have vivid memories of my mum and dad cajoling and insisting I eat what was served on my plate but all the while the food I did take in went round and round in my mouth because I was unable to swallow it.

I know that it was with love and concern that they insisted that I sit at the table until I cleaned my plate but mealtimes were a tense battle ground for the three of us.

Because of my parent's concern we had visits to the family doctor and then to an eminent paediatrician to find out why I wouldn't eat. The paediatrician's advice to my parents was:

"Don't worry. She is growing and thriving and is not sick. Just relax, keep offering good food and eventually she will eat it."

This was sound advice from a wise and experienced man way back then.

And it worked!

Each of my three children went through the typically picky toddler stages and at times we, as parents, became exasperated. With memories of how stressful mealtimes were for me as a child we tried to keep our cool and persisted in offering healthy family food. Now as young adults they have very sophisticated palates, love trying new foods and flavours, and all love cooking what they call real food.

Some degree of food rejection or pickiness is fairly normal behaviour for a lot of toddlers and pre-schoolers. It is only a phase and it will pass. More importantly, don't take it personally. It does not mean that you are a poor parent or a bad cook!

So here are some hints and suggestions I have gleaned from my own childhood experiences, my experiences as a parent of three delightful children, and as a naturopath and nutrition medicine consultant with over 28 years of experience treating children and their families.

Why Do Children Become Picky With Food? Fussy Eating Facts

There are very real and legitimate reasons that children become so fussy with food. And it is not just to annoy and frustrate parents or to be obstinate. Yes I know you were thinking it. I've thought it too!

Understanding those reasons, the science behind them and the sources of a child's picky eating habits will go a long way in helping you work around the problem and, when possible, enable your child to eat more healthily and broaden their tastes.

Picky Eaters are Born That Way

Really? Yes really!

There are definite developmental and biological reasons. For example, toddlers will be just beginning to learn to distinguish between what is food and what is not. You will have noticed that babies and toddlers keenly explore their world with their mouth. They are learning about taste, texture and that, in spite of the interesting sound a toy makes when biting it, it's not actually food. Multiply those thoughts by the fact that they are also learning what foods are safe.

Innate Survival Tactics

There are two main underlying reasons that children can be so specific about the foods they will eat.

- *Children generally prefer sweet rather than bitter tastes.*
- *Children dislike or may be afraid of trying new foods or new tastes.*

Science suggests that both of these are rooted in basic survival techniques.

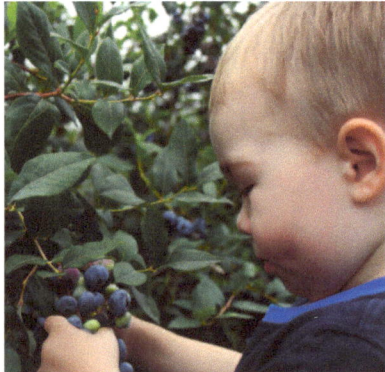

In so many ways we are all still 'wired' like our prehistoric ancestors. A dislike of bitter foods can be seen as a protective mechanism to avoid eating things that are poisonous. For example: A toddler in prehistoric times, when exploring their world, would be less likely to ingest a poisonous food due to its bitter taste. Children are naturally attracted to sweet foods such as fruits which are safe and energy and nutrient rich. Mother's milk which is also 'safe' is relatively sweet. It may take years for kids to develop a taste for sour or bitter foods like some vegetables.

This suspicion or dislike of new foods is technically known as food neophobia, or fear of eating new things. It is usually about the age of 2 years that most traditional societies cease breastfeeding and the child is less dependent on their mother for food. Avoiding unfamiliar foods is an innate way of keeping safe as a young child, when left to their own devices, having no real way of knowing what is or is not safe to eat.

So it is very natural for children, especially toddlers and pre-schoolers to be wary of new and unfamiliar foods.

Developmental and Growth Rates

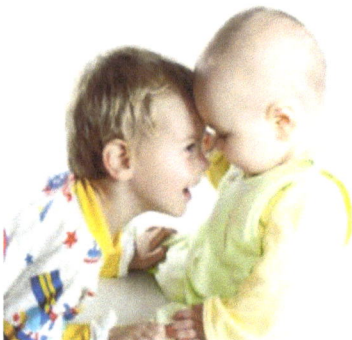

There are also developmental reasons why young children have variable appetites and often become picky with food. As a baby your child was fed constantly and grew rapidly. By their first birthday they will have probably tripled their birth weight.

Toddlers and young children grow at a much slower rate than when they were babies so their requirements for food are a little less than many parents expect. As well, they are usually too busy learning about their world to sit still for anything, even to eat.

Children's limited and sporadic appetites are also affected by their growth cycles or growth spurts and by variations in activity. It is quite common for children to be hungry one day or for a few days in a row and then picky the next.

They are more likely to eat better (and their requirements will be greater) during periods of more rapid growth.

Some young children and fussy eaters may do better having most of their food as frequent nutrient dense snacks rather than fewer larger meals.

The secret is to nurture and guide a child's developing food choices in the same way we nurture their physical and emotional development – little by little, in the same way we help them to walk, to read, swim or ride a bike.

Physiological and Other Reasons

The reasons why children may reject foods can be many and varied and will differ with each child. Try to understand the possible reasons for your child's fussiness. Is it due to innate issues, due to particular habits being created around food initially or is there some other underlying condition?

For instance, research at Brown University in the US showed that damage to the taste system from ear infections and tonsillectomies alters taste perception and does have an effect on food preferences. Certainly in my naturopathic practice, the majority of children I see with picky or poor eating behaviour are found to have an underlying health issue of some type. This might be a subclinical chronic respiratory infection, allergy or intolerance or nutrient deficiencies that can be both the cause and effect of less than ideal health and picky eating behaviours.

A deficiency of the minerals zinc and iron are commonly behind these types of problems. Zinc specifically will influence both smell and taste. If you can't smell or taste food it is then very difficult to have any enjoyment or interest in food. Refer to appendix 2 for more information on these minerals.

Below is a list of other possible reasons for your child's fussiness:

- *Is unwell from a cold, ear infection, sore throat, swollen tonsils and/or adenoids*
- *Is teething and has sore gums*
- *Is too tired to eat or over tired*
- *Is emotionally upset*
- *Is put off by lack of routine and familiarity surrounding mealtimes*
- *Is suffering some digestive discomfort or reflux*
- *Is constipated*
- *Is suffering from allergies or sensitivities*
- *Is suffering from specific nutrient insufficiencies such as iron and zinc which impact on his food choices and food behaviour.*
- *Has poor muscle tone and difficulty with oral motor skills such as chewing*
- *Has trouble managing the meal e.g. problems chewing or using fork etc*
- *Peers and other family members reject the food*
- *The amount he is expected to eat is too large*
- *Is already full from snacks*
- *Dislikes the appearance and/or smell of the food being offered*
- *Is increasing the ability to exercise independence and control and is testing boundaries (especially around 2yrs!!)*
- *The eating environment has become stressful for them*
- *Has an autistic spectrum or other neurological disorder.*

Remember too that little ones are not just little adults but have a different approach to eating and different appetites. They are also likely to dawdle over meals or may be too busy and excited about what they are doing to settle to food so quickly lose interest or become distracted very easily.

Physiologically a child's gut, brain and immune system are not yet fully developed. Each of these systems and the interrelationship between them is especially vulnerable to imbalances. Their gut lining is still rather leaky and liver detoxification ability is not mature so children are not capable of handling toxins from foods or their environment effectively. This can have a significant impact on their overall health as well as mood and eating behaviour.

How Long Will It Last?

As adults we have grown to accept new foods through repeated exposure to them and by modelling on what those around us (parents, siblings, relatives, and friends) ate plus developing positive associations with those foods. The more exposure and positive associations developed regarding a food the more it will become acceptable. I can see this clearly now in my own association with food. Foods that I disliked or wouldn't even taste as a child are now included in my diet and greatly enjoyed.

The key here is to guide your picky kid (no matter what age) through their experiences of and exposures to foods just as you would support their physical development such as your toddler's attempts to walk or learning to ride a bike.

Usually toddlers who have been picky will become more accepting of their food when they reach around three or four years of age.

For some it may last up to school age and beyond. In most cases picky eating behaviour will change once the underlying causes have been addressed. So, given the right environment, the majority of children will, for the most part, leave this phase behind them as they grow and mature physically and emotionally.

Key points

- ✓ *Picky eating can vary from occasionally fussy with food to extreme selective eating behaviours.*
- ✓ *Some fussiness and pickiness is a very common but normal developmental phase in toddlerhood.*
- ✓ *A large number of parents have concerns about their child's eating. You are certainly not alone.*
- ✓ *Picky and fussy eating may be due to underlying issues such as illness, developmental delays and stress. It is important to investigate and deal with underlying issues.*

CHAPTER 2
How Do I Cope With My Picky Eater?

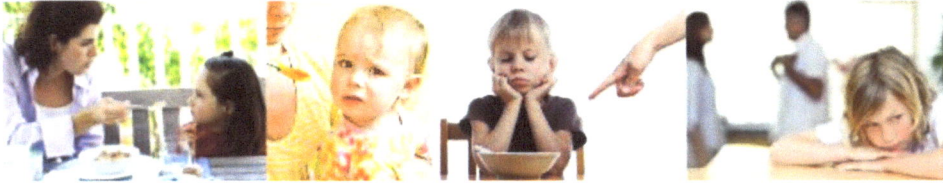

"Parents should control the what, when and where of feeding and give the child autonomy with respect to choosing what and how much to eat" – Ellyn Satter

Calmly !

At least keep as calm as possible, however difficult and frustrating this may be. Dealing with an extremely picky eater or one that refuses to eat can be one of the most frustrating and anxiety producing situations a parent can face. Some parents even feel that they are somehow to blame and are fearful that their child will become ill or will not grow and thrive.

In my practice I have seen many families who were in this situation with their picky eater. After assessing and dealing with underlying health issues we have implemented many of the strategies I'm outlining for you in this book. The outcome has been happy healthy children who eat well and enjoy a variety of nutritious foods.

When it comes down to it, the fact is you can't force your child to eat, but you can give them every encouragement and opportunity to take in their basic nutrient requirements.

Ensure that there is only nutrient dense, healthy foods in your fridge or pantry and ensure that these are easily accessible for the whole family.

Gently take charge and don't shy away from insisting on good eating habits. It is important to let your child know that you insist on this because you love them and want them to be well, happy and healthy.

Be as calm, relaxed and nonchalant as possible and try not to focus too much on the picky behaviour. Focus instead of the more positive aspects of your relationship with your child.

Don't Rush

Within reason, let your child take time with meals and allow them to eat slowly. Young children are naturally slow eaters and fussy, picky eaters even more so! Remember, it takes up to 20 minutes for the brain to get the message that the body has had enough to eat.

Eating slowly is a good habit to encourage. Eating slowly aids digestion and reduces the likelihood of overeating. Eating should be a pleasurable and social experience.

Start Early

Habits are formed early, so stick to your guns and encourage your child to experience a variety of foods encompassing a range of flavours, colours and textures so that they get used to trying new things.

Try to avoid bad habits forming. Some pickiness with food can be merely a habit and once formed, habits can be hard to break.

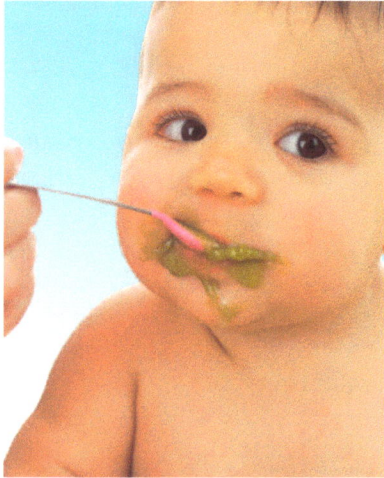

Research shows that children offered a variety of healthy foods and different tastes from the start tend to be less picky with food and are more likely to follow a healthy diet later in life. An eight year study of 70 mothers and babies at the University of Tennessee, published in 2002, confirmed that food preferences are established as early as two years of age, and that eight year olds usually like the same foods they did when they were four.

As most experts agree that the period before age 2 is critical for establishing healthy eating it is important to offer your child a variety of colourful, nutrient dense family foods at each meal from an early age.

Take action at the first sign of picky behaviour. Employ some of the suggestions here to break any troublesome habits forming.

Be a Good Role Model

When it comes to healthy eating, the best thing you can do as a parent is to be a good role model. Don't expect your child to eat foods that you won't.

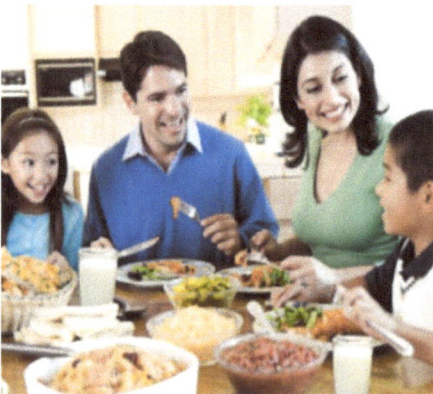

What your child learns about food begins with you. You may not realise it but you are continually educating your child about food, especially during the first 10 years or so of their life.

Research has shown that most picky eaters grow out of this stage when they are ready and particularly where the closest role models (parents) have healthy eating habits for them to emulate.

Most children want to be "mini you", be just like mum and dad. Most parents notice, comment on and smile at imitative behaviours such as talking on a pretend mobile phone like mum or dad BUT have you made the connection between imitation of your own eating habits and your child's eating habits?

Children are very keen observers of what significant adults in their lives are doing. As well as parents, this will include grandparents, extended family members, family friends and even older brothers and sisters.

Research indicates it is more the modelling of parental eating habits that leads to better long term nutrition.

Key points

- ✓ *You can't fake good role modelling, so you have to do it with foods you like.*
- ✓ *Frequency is key. The more often you eat nutritious whole foods, the more likely your child will do the same.*
- ✓ *It does not work immediately; it needs practice like developing any skill.*
- ✓ *Modelling does not involve pressure, suggesting or cajoling. It is passive. The more you suggest or persuade, the less likely your picky kid will want to try a new food.*
- ✓ *Concentrate on preparing and enjoying nutritious foods in the ways you like and let your child absorb your attitudes and behaviours to the foods just as they will with other aspects of life such as your attitudes to friendships or sports for instance.*

Here are some important questions to consider

- ☐ *Do I eat regular meals – breakfast, lunch and dinner? If you don't, how can you expect your child to do so?*
- ☐ *Do I always eat healthy nutrient dense fresh foods? If you expectdon't, how can you expect your child to?*
- ☐ *Do I pick at food and not eat particular vegetables? Your child will mimic this. If mum or dad is a picky eater and isn't willing to eat the new foods, neither will the child.*
- ☐ *Where do I eat meals? In front of the TV? At the kitchen bench? On the run driving to work?*
- ☐ *Does my family sit together and enjoy the majority of breakfasts and evening meals together?*
- ☐ *Do I share the same meal as my child or do I expect them to eat something differen?.*

Take a little time to think carefully about these questions and about ways in which you might become a better role model to help your picky eater.

The key here is to show rather than tell your child how to eat well. Your actions will speak louder than words.

What your child learns from you in their early years will impact on their health and nutrition habits for the rest of their life.

Be Persistent

IF AT FIRST YOU DON'T SUCCEED, TRY, TRY AGAIN! If at first you don't succeed try, try and try again. Be consistent, firm and don't give up. Use the same tactics at every meal.

Resolve to be committed to your plan for at least 30 days. You can't just try for a few days and then give up because it gets a bit tough. And it certainly can get tough!

Avoid feeding any negative or troublesome picky eating behaviour with your attention. Better not to argue, cajole, negotiate, plead or get drawn into discussions or deals or you will never get on top of the problem behaviour. Resolve is your key from the outset.

It is common for children to go on and off foods so remain committed to your grand plan. Continue to offer a wide variety of healthy family foods with different colours and textures along with some of what you know they like or whatever is the most recent fad food.

Even if a meal is rejected, at least your picky kid is still being exposed to food that will form part of their diet later on. When a food is rejected once don't be afraid to offer it again and again. A food is more likely to be accepted if it is familiar and tastes can change quickly. Research shows that it may need to be presented up to 15 times before it is accepted. So you can see that perseverance and patience are essential!

Believe it or not, not every meal with your picky kid has to turn into a fight over food.

Avoid turning meals into a power struggle. It doesn't help. The constant pressure can make your child more resistant to eating and may even result in the development of negative feelings about food. Parent-child conflicts over eating, excessive parent control and stressful mealtimes have been noted as risk factors in the development of eating disorders.

Oh boy! I can remember vividly the stress and drama at mealtimes with my parents and the bargaining, cajoling and tactics to get me to eat. Luckily something eventually changed. Was it me or was it my parent's approach, or perhaps a bit of both. But, thankfully there was a shift and I seem to have managed well as a teen and an adult.

Toddlers in particular are just starting to express their independence, finding their own power and love to get a reaction.

For toddlers, food refusal can be a way of exerting this new found power and can quickly learn that they can trigger a parental reaction by refusing food. Avoid mealtime battles becoming a habit. When they refuse, fling food or tantrum, keep calm and matter of fact and if possible (as long as they are safe) walk away. If the food isn't eaten in a reasonable time, take it away and re-offer it later if need be.

Keeping calm, nonchalant and consistent in your approach will not be reinforcing the negative behaviour and for the most part that behaviour will probably stop no matter what the age of your child.

Avoid being emotionally attached to your child's eating behaviour. Children will pick up on your anxiety. They may then come to associate meal time with stress or may even play on your anxiety to get their way with the meal.

I know you probably dread every mealtime and the dramas that they usually entail. That is understandable, but take it easy; you won't be able to change a picky eater's habits overnight. Take small, easy but consistent steps. Start by addressing just one meal a day and make it as nutritious as possible.

Put the food on your child's plate, but if it stays there, don't push or demand that they eat it.

Don't stress over it.

Offering just some limited choices regarding a meal may be enough to avert a power struggle. For example offer some choices that don't really matter such as, "Do you want to have the white plate or the yellow plate?" or "Would you like peas or beans today?"

Keep eating and make mealtimes a pleasurable experience for the whole family.

Never Reward or Punish With Food

Using food as reward or punishment may give the message that food equals love and approval. This is not a good thought for young children and could pose difficulties if carried on into later life setting up an unhealthy relationship with food.

Certainly never make dessert of sweets the reward for eating their as this sets up the belief that dessert is more valuable than vegetables and whole primary foods.

Instead, use rewards that are unrelated to food such as extra hugs and praise, a special new book or extra stories at bedtime, trips to a favourite playground or park. Focusing on the good behaviour encourages your child to keep eating well.

Don't Fuss If Food Goes Uneaten

Try to ignore poor eating habits and complaints such as "Yuck!", or "There is no way I'm eating that" however hard and upsetting this may be. Cajoling, forcing or coercing a child to eat is counterproductive and not advisable. In fact it can have the reverse effect and could lead to mealtimes becoming a type of power game.

Children can be put off their food when eating becomes stressful. Take it gently.

If your little one throws a tantrum at the table try not to focus on it too much. Make sure they are safe but reduce eye contact and divert your attention elsewhere.

If they refuse to eat, end the meal. Don't make them sit there for hours. This only adds to the stress and tension and is counterproductive in the long term.

Remove the plate when they refuse to eat any more. If your child is really hungry later offer the meal again, a healthy snack such as vegetable sticks with a dip of hommos or guacamole or a sandwich with filling of some of the rejected food mashed with nut butter.

Don't offer sweet treats.

If the food still goes uneaten, to avoid waste, present it again later in a different form.

Praise, Praise, Praise and Be Positive

The road to healthy, varied eating may be a long one for you and your picky eater. Just the slightest acceptance of a new food after weeks or months will be worth a cheer.

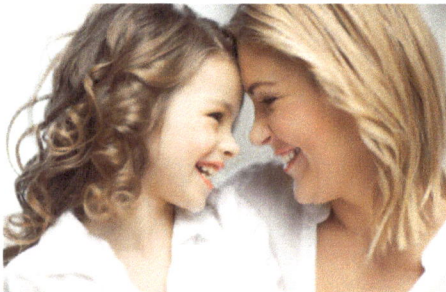

Even if your child has just one nibble or a small mouthful, congratulate and praise them. If they have just tried something more than previously, they have achieved something – no matter how small. If they played with it, smelled it, licked it, chewed it and swallowed it or even spat it out, focus on and praise them for what they have done. This is a major victory!

Focus your praise on what they are doing *for themselves* (not for you) and how good that food will be for them to grow, be strong and healthy and achieve whatever they idolise.

Leave whatever they have not done unmentioned and certainly never punish for what wasn't achieved.

Use positive language – **if you say it, it will become true**. Talk about their good choices and little victories in a way that encourages them to make those choices again. Very simply, re-enforce the positive and ignore the negative.

Key points

- ✓ Stay calm and don't rush your child
- ✓ Introduce a variety of food early
- ✓ Be a good role model
- ✓ Be persistent but firm without too much fuss
- ✓ Never reward or punish with food
- ✓ Praise even the slightest progress.

Try a Little Peer Pressure

Peer pressure can be a great tactic.

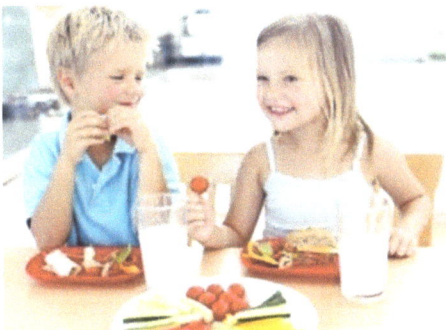

Invite other children of a similar age or just slightly older (especially if they are good eaters!) around for a meal.

Studies show that children often copy their peers at mealtime, so if they see their friends eating something or eating a full plate of food, they are more likely want to join in and try those foods themselves.

Let the others set the example.

And praise them for what they attempt!

Write down some actions you can take right now to deal with your little picky eater.

....
....
....
....
....
....
....
....
....
....
....
....
....
....
....

CHAPTER 3
MEALTIME STRATEGIES

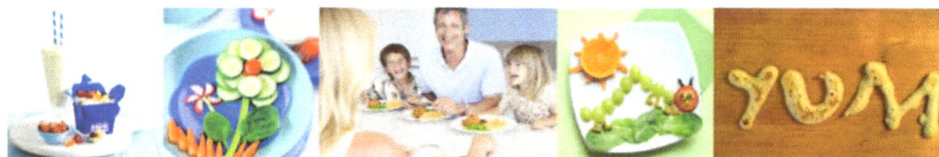

Understanding certain aspects of eating behaviours and using strategies such as involving your child in decisions about their food can go a long way toward reducing your own anxiety about your little one's food intake and at the same time help your child engage with food in a healthy way. Also involve them in shopping for food, food preparation, and assist them in growing some of their own.

Autonomy, Independence and Inconsistencies

"I do it my own self!" Sound familiar?

This was my son's favourite sentence as he exerted his new-found toddler independence.

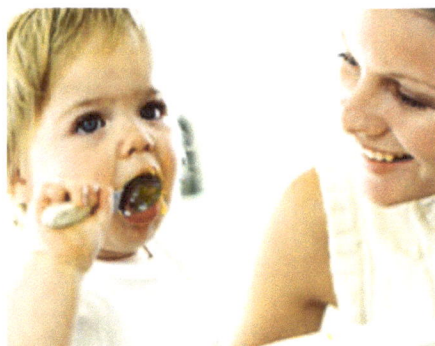

I think this phrase epitomises all aspects of toddlerhood and particularly their eating. Once my little boy found that he could put his shoes or shorts on himself that was the only way it could be done. He also didn't want help from mum or dad when it came to eating. He fussed and fretted at being spoon fed but just loved feeding himself with finger foods. Having learned this with the first child, we offered our daughters finger foods early and had a lot fewer hassles at meal time.

Young children don't have much ownership or say in too many things. When given the opportunity to do something for themselves or be involved in picking out a particular vegetable or fruit for a meal it really gives them a feeling of worthiness and autonomy.

Give in to a few demands or preferences. This will help them feel that they have a little more control. It reinforces that you care about their opinion and want to make things they like.

Here are some ideas to try.

- Whenever practical, involve your child in the food choices, meal preparations and serving. They will enjoy taking ownership of some decisions and will be more likely to eat the food if they have some involvement and connection to it.

- Involve them in organising the shopping list, shopping for and selecting the food as well as its preparation. Make a game of it. For example, ask them to find their favourite red, green or orange vegetable or to choose which beans or nuts they would like to add to a salad. Ask what they would like for dinner. Do your best to accommodate.

- Even a three year old can be involved in washing vegetables or choosing vegetables for dinner. Then praise their good work with the whole family at mealtime.

- Older children especially love setting the table, finding the placemats, or getting flowers for the table.This makes them feel special and that they have contributed.

- Allow your really fussy eater to explore and play with food. This allows them to explore and experience different textures through the tactile system and might lead to a better relationship with their food. A hypersensitive child may find it "safer"and less threatening to check out textures with their hand first rather than their mouth.

- Encourage self-feeding and exploration of food. Babies and young children initially learn about their world via their mouth and touch. Being actively involved in eating, rather than sitting passively receiving food, will encourage them to take more of an interest in the food they are being served. Don't worry too much about mess. Spread an old sheet, plastic or newspaper under their eating area so the mess can be disposed of easily afterward. Allow even your very young child to have their own bowl containing some finger food and their own spoon. Finger foods will allow a toddler their desired independence.

- Also encourage your child to feed themselves by having healthy snacks readily available and easily accessible so they can self-regulate food intake to some extent. Supervise their eating and encourage them to eat sitting down, not running around. Provide them with their own child sized table and chairs with the food available on a tray or in containers on the table.

- Keep choices manageable. While allowing your child to make choices within the range of healthy food options you offer, keep the options limited to only 2 or 3 different things so they don't become too confused or overwhelmed as to what to choose to eat. For example, ask simply, "Do you want beans or broccoli for dinner?"

- Be prepared for some inconsistency in what and how much your child is willing to eat. This can vary daily. Small children, especially in the 1 to 4 year age group, often have fads. For example they may eat only fruit one day and only vegetables or red things the next or eat lots one day and virtually nothing the next. They may want to feed themselves one day and for you to feed them the next. Go with these whims to some extent and don't take it personally. In this case aim for a nutritionally balanced week rather than a balanced day.

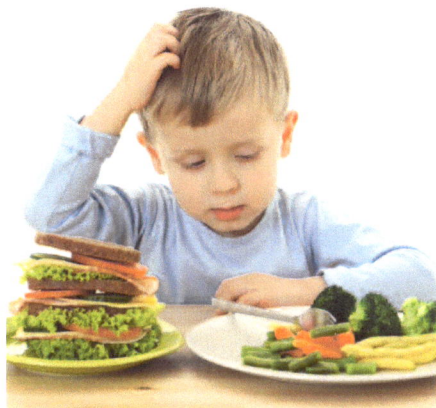

- Children can also go through periods of having very set ideas about everything, including food. For example it may become of upmost and dire importance as to the order that foods are placed on a plate or on a sandwich. Again, go with the flow. This too is a passing developmental phase. They are just learning about the order of things in their world.

- Involve your child in growing their own foods. Some vegetables grow well even in pots on a deck or veranda if there is no garden space. Try cherry or tear drop tomatoes, baby lettuce, carrots, peas, beans and various herbs. Bean and seed sprouts are also very easy to grow in containers in the kitchen and will provide a nutrient dense snack. Even toddlers and very young children can be involved with a little guidance from mum and dad.

Happy Family Mealtime Works its Magic

Twenty-first century family life can be hectic. There is always so much on – mothers' group, play group, Jimboree, swimming lessons, music lessons and more as well as parents' work schedule and commitments.

Do you always sit down for meals as a family?

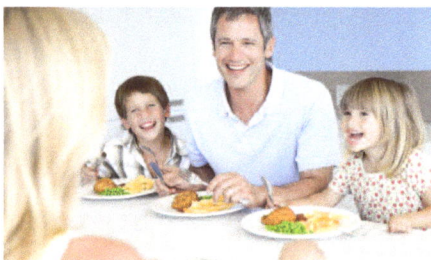

Research is proving that eating as a family has a positive impact on just about all aspects of children's lives, from general health, to school performance and social behaviour. It has emphasised that it is the actual togetherness, the sitting down face to face and the sharing of food even more than the type of actual food eaten that is most beneficial.

The benefit is by just being with you, by watching how and what you eat and talking with you. This is how, by modelling, they will absorb everything from social skills, good table manners, to good eating habits to the very nutrients from the food.

For picky eaters, family meals are essential.

- Mealtimes need to be a family occasion. Togetherness at mealtimes is as valuable for your child's overall development as it is for all family relationships. It is a great opportunity to develop social skills and as an opportunity to emulate mum and dad and their healthy eating habits. If you are enjoying nutrient dense, whole, real foods together this will assist them to develop an understanding of good nutrition.

- Young children should not eat alone. At the very least sit down with your child while he or she is eating and perhaps have your own small portion of food.

- Family meals should be an occasion - a family oriented, stress free, happy and enjoyable social occasion. Above all try to make mealtimes fun – whether your child eats or not. Have a chat and enjoy each other's company. Even if they don't eat everything today, or tomorrow, they may do next week!

- Turn the TV off. Regularly eating in front of the television is distracting and often results in picky eaters eating even less. The meal and those eating it should be the centre of attention, not the TV, a toy or a book

- Don't sweat the small stuff. It doesn't really matter if your lovingly prepared broccoli was eaten or not. Keep the focus on the sitting down together. That is what matters most.

Put Fun on the Menu

Keep mealtimes and food fun. Be creative.

It's interesting how food made into shapes can tempt even the most sceptical eaters. Mashed potato made into a snowman for example will have much more appeal than just a spoonful on the plate even though it is exactly the same food.

Colour their World

Use brightly coloured plates, bowls, cutlery, table cloths and placemats. Maybe use the theme of a favourite story or cartoon character. On the other hand, a colourful selection of foods on a white plate may be more appealing to some children.

Picky Kids to Budding Chefs

Encourage your little one to invent new "recipes" and help prepare new snacks, sandwiches, trail mixes or smoothies. Then name the dish they've helped create after them, for example - "Sam's Super Sandwich", "Madeline's Marvellous Fruit Salad", or "Max's Funny Face Rissoles". Make a big deal of serving and presenting the dish as their own special creation.

Food Art

Fruit on a plate becomes pretty butterflies

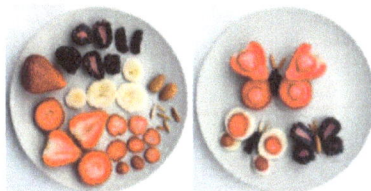

- Try some food art or veggie art. This can be great fun and your little one can develop their creativity. Use cookie cutters to cut and form different shapes. On a meat patty or a star or 'man' of bread or cheese, try peas for eyes, a piece of carrot for a nose & grated cheese for hair. Children's books and the internet are great places for ideas. I have listed some useful sites in the references and reading section.

- Use a pancake or thin biscuit mixture in a turkey baster or squeeze top plastic bottle to pipe shapes, letters, or your child's name onto a frying pan or baking sheet. Children love these as snacks or to accompany their meals.

- Your little chef themselves may love to shape a mince (finely grated or mashed/pureed vegetables already added) or patty mixture into balls, hamburgers, sausages etc using pieces of cut vegetables to add faces, make clowns, houses, or boats etc. Adding some long grain cooked rice can make these into hedgehogs. Just add the eyes, nose and whiskers. My children loved doing this and came up with some amazing creations. There was often a bit of a mess but they always ate their creations happily!

- Imaginative presentation of a meal may make all the difference. Try to choose different coloured and textured foods and arrange them in an attractive pattern. Or thread fruit or cubes of cheese and baby tomatoes onto paddle pop sticks. See how much more appealing pieces of fruit can be when arranged for fun.

- Discuss the foods your child selects to eat in a happy way and avoid commenting on how it might taste. Comment instead on the shape, colour or 'function' of what he is eating. For example, "Oh my goodness, are you eating the clown's nose, now how will he smell things?" or "Wow! You ate the whole of the little tree. That is going to make you really big and strong like daddy /so you can swim a long, long way".

Names and Rhymes

Call finger foods playful names. For example green balls (grapes), red balls (cherry tomatoes), wheels (rounds of carrot), swords (carrot or celery sticks), building blocks (diced cheese), ants on a log (celery sticks with nut butter or cottage cheese & topped with sultanas or currants), traffic lights (pieces of red, orange, and greenfruit on a cracker).

Engage your picky kid in singing songs and rhymes related to various foods. Here are a few examples.

- *Cherries, cherries, ruby red, want to try one? Go ahead.*
- *I'm full of seeds, my flesh is green. I have the prickliest skin you've ever seen. Kiwi, kiwi is my name.*
- *Monkeys eat me, kids do too. Gorillas love me, how 'bout you?*
- *The incredible, edible egg.*
- *Tomatoes make your cheeks go red, carrots make you jump ahead, spinach makes you very strong, peas will make you dance along! Eat your veggies every day to make you happy every day.*
- *Apples are red, berries are blue, pears are sweet and they're all good for you*

Change the Venue

A picnic at a park or at the beach can be a treat but you can even try a picnic on the veranda, in the back yard or just on a cloth or mat on the kitchen floor. Most children love the idea of a picnic and it creates novelty around mealtime. Prepare the food in a slightly different "picnic" finger food form and it is more likely to be at least tried but probably eaten happily.

Follow a Theme

Link Foods to Your Child's Interests

Basing a meal on a theme, such as a favourite cartoon character, game, book or season, can be quite successful. One of the mums that I see in my clinic did this.

Her fussy little man was mad about dinosaurs so she found a dinosaur cookie cutter to cut some foods into dinosaur shapes, used broccoli "trees" sitting in mashed potato as a dinosaur's forest. All this was set on a colourful plate and placemat all with the dinosaur theme and guess what! As long as his food was associated with his dinosaur passion, it was eaten without any fuss!

Make foods into different shapes (use cookie cutters) or make associations with the food that might capture your child's imagination relating to dinosaurs, robots, cars, fairies, rabbit, "The Wiggles" and the like.

For instance carrot slices could be the wheels of a car, broccoli flowerets can be dinosaur food or the tree beside the doll's house, thin strips of carrot could be a wire to give the robot power. Even thin slices of meat, chicken or fish can be cut into favourite shapes with a cookie cutter.

Place mats, dishes, plates and cutlery could also contribute to the theme or interest.

You probably won't have to go to this trouble for ever and you may not even get your child to actually like the food but at least it will increase the likelihood of them trying it.

Introducing New Foods

Introducing new foods can be a challenge in some families and for some children.

First impressions count!

You rarely have more than one chance to impress. The way a new food is first presented will be of vital importance so try to make it the most pleasant encounter possible.

Try some of the following hints to ease the way

- *A new food may be more readily accepted if your child is relaxed and not too tired.*

- *Presenting a new food as "a special treat" may make your child more inclined to eat it – or at least try it.*

- *Always serve a little of at least one food that your child likes or is the current fad in addition to the few food. They then know there is at least something on their plate that they will enjoy.*

- *Include just a small portion (maybe only 1 teaspoonful) of a new food and serve everyone at the table with the same food. Make sure the whole family participates and eats the food.*

- *Involve your child in the preparation of the new food. For example get them to count enough carrot sticks for everyone, put some on each plate or stir the fruit salad.*

- *Combine foods that you know your child likes with others that are untried or previously rejected.*

- *Introduce new foods slowly, one at a time. Too many new tastes and foods may be overwhelming to a small child. Also, this way you will notice if there is any reaction or allergy to a new food.*

- *Some children are more likely to accept a new food if it is separate. For others, it is more likely to be eaten if the new food is mixed in with the favourite food. Respect their preferences and go with it.*

- *Offer a new food in a texture that you know your child likes, for example crunchy, smooth and creamy or chunky. See the 'Favourite Textures' section below for more ideas.*

- *Encourage your child to try a variety of foods but if they have tried a food and don't like it, don't force the issue too much. Everyone, including you, has foods they like and dislike. Keep serving the food regularly and don't fuss if it isn't eaten. Over time they may be willing to try it again and may accept it or reject it again.*

- *Some children may be more likely to try a new food if they have the option of not having to swallow it. Show them how to carefully spit the food into a tissue or napkin if they don't want to eat it.*

Children develop differently and at different paces. Try not to compare with others.

Timing, Routine and Small Tummies

Children thrive on routine. Some form of routine may provide a picky, fussy eater with some predictability. Very young children in particular find comfort in familiarity and predictability.

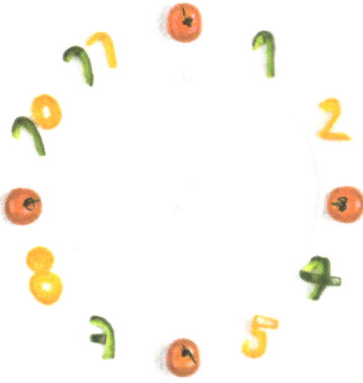

Keep main meals and snack times at roughly the same time each day. Children have a strong need for rituals and for what feels familiar whether it is a bedtime routine, meal time or a favourite plate.

Set up regular habits for eating and make sure that your child understands what is expected of them when they eat.

- Offer the evening meal at a realistic time. Children are usually hungry around 4.30 or 5pm. Offer the main evening meal then. It is more likely to be eaten.

- A healthy snack or a small snack portion of the adult meal can be offered when the whole family sits down to dinner later. In summer, an ice block or pudding made from a protein and fruit smoothie mix is an ideal early afternoon snack or after dinner treat.

- I found this strategy really helpful with my three when they were little. They were hungriest in the afternoon after school or kindergarten so I offered a fairly substantial nutrient dense, protein and vegetable meal or "snack" at that time rather than have them fill up on other snack food. They still took part in the family evening meal but had slightly smaller helpings. For us, this resulted in much less discussions and arguments around food.

- A toddler may need some quiet time before meals so they can calm down a little and have time to divert their attention from play time to eating time. A table setting and hand washing routine may help with this.

- Try not to get too hung up on the time of day your child eats or how much they eat at each sitting.

- Don't worry if you child decides on upside down meals sometimes. If they occasionally want fruit and cereal for dinner and meat and vegetables for breakfast, it doesn't matter as long as both meals are nutrient dense. The difference between breakfast, lunch and dinner has little meaning to small children.

- Don't expect your child to eat well or very much if they are over tired or unwell.

- Respect tiny tummies. A young child's stomach is roughly just the size of their fist so serve just small portions initially and then top it up with more later if they want more. Smaller portions are less off-putting to little tummies.

- Finger foods are also popular and will allow a toddler some of their desired independence.

- If your little one is struggling to eat what you have served on their plate, separate out a small portion for them to eat. For example, two bite sized pieces of meat, one bean and two carrot circles.

- Small and frequent nutrient dense mini meals can work well for some picky, fussy kids. Small bodies have small tummies and fast metabolisms. They don't need much to get full so may only want small amounts at a time but get hungry again quickly. Just a small amount of food on the plate will be far less intimidating and more likely to be eaten, especially if it is a new food.

- Children need to eat frequently to sustain their high energy levels and rapid growth. Your toddler or young child may do better with six or more smaller meals throughout the day that will maintain optimum blood sugar levels and keep the grumpiness, pickiness and tantrums at bay. Every parent knows that a hungry child is generally not a happy or co-operative child.

- Older children need three proper meals daily with two well-spaced nutritious snacks.

- Don't just regard snacks as a "fill in" between meals. For really difficult eaters, snacks are a great opportunity to boost healthy food intake as nutrient dense mini meals. Be prepared and have these available for your child to access when they need to.

- Stop all snacks and drinks at least one hour before mealtime. A hungry kid, even a picky one, is more likely to eat what your present at mealtime.

Make it Easily Accessible

Children are natural grazers. While it will suit some better to have specific times for snacks and meals, for others, having a choice of healthy and varied foods is easily accessible and within their reach, they will eat better when able to help themselves.

- For toddlers and very young children try offering a nibble tray containing some bite sized portions of nutritious foods in a compartmentalised dish or tray. Place this in an easy to reach spot such as their own little table, where they can have a nibble from time to time in their busy play. Also make sure that there is always plenty of pure water available for drinking.

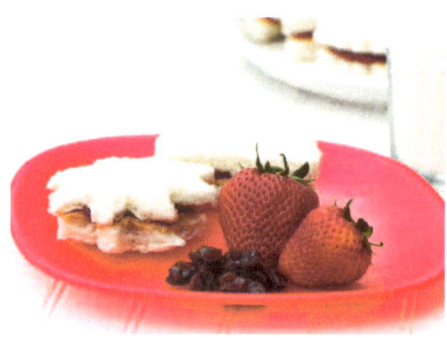

- Rather than storing fruit and vegetables out of sight in the crisper after shopping chop and prepare some to keep in see through containers in the refrigerator, on the kitchen bench or table. I would suggest a couple of small pots of natural yoghurt, a container of grapes, strawberries, blueberries, mandarin segments, cherry tomatoes, carrot and celery sticks, and sliced capsicum. Have these at your child's eye level and easy reach for their convenience. Also have a container of filtered water or a yummy healthy smoothie for them to sip from time to time. This works especially well for older children.

- Be ready to go at a moments notice with Snacky Bags. Keep a supply of ready to eat fruit, vegetables or healthy snacks in small containers or zip lock plastic bags in the refrigerator to grab for outings. Having a special sticker or their name on it is handy if you have more than one child. They then have ownership of their Snacky Bag and there will be fewer squabbles. This enables children to eat when they are hungry, an important step in developing a healthy attitude toward food.

Respect Your Child's Tastes, Preferences and Appetite

Know when to let go. This can be really hard but it is important to respect your child when they say they are not hungry or really dislike a particular food. It does no one any good to force your child to eat. Most young children will only eat when they are hungry and remember that it doesn't take much to fill a tiny tummy.

Talk to your child to establish their likes and dislikes. We all have preferences and some foods we dislike. Allowing some choice will help them feel more in control of their diet.

Of course you want to keep encouraging them to eat a variety of foods but if they have tried it and say they don't like it then respect that. Keep offering that food from time to time. Eventually they may try it again and decide they like it after all!

In the meantime, try serving the disliked food in a different way. For example, if they don't like red meat, serve it finely ground (a food processor does this well) in a vegetable laden pasta sauce or as vegetable laden baby meat balls (with faces!). Alternatively you could substitute other foods of similar nutritional value and make-up such as lamb, pork, chicken or egg plus nut and seed meal.

The same goes for preferred foods. If your picky kid will only eat a narrow range of foods, try adding a twist to introduce a little variety. For example, if they are hooked on peanut butter sandwiches, try offering almond or a mixed nut butter sandwich. Alternatively, try peanut butter in celery stalks topped with currants making "ants on a log".

Engage Your Picky Eater Using a Reward Chart

Have you tried using a reward chart to help engage your fussy eater? This can be helpful even for children who just need some encouragement to try something new or to teach basic nutrition concepts.

Behaviour incentive charts have been proven to be effective tools for eliciting positive behavioural and eating behaviours in children. They work particularly well for children aged from about 2 or 3 through to about 8 years.

Every time your child takes a bite of something they place a sticker on the chart. Placing a star or a sticker on the chart shows your child that they are being rewarded for trying hard with that behaviour. With your continual praise and encouragement and their continued success, not only will your child's eating behaviour and nutrition improve but their self-esteem will flourish.

The reward chart will work best when:

- *First of all choose very specific and measurable goals that are appropriate for the age and developmental level of your child. For example, for your picky eater just to put a new food in their mouth or your child to try a new food or a specific coloured vegetable such as a green bean.*

- *Discuss the idea with your child and come up with and agree on a list of privileges or rewards. For example agree on some short term or daily rewards if they reach a certain goal or number of "points" (e.g. an extra or special story at bedtime, watching a favourite TV show) and then when they have achieved a certain number of stickers or "points", a bigger weekly reward such as a new toy, book or a trip to the movies.*

- *Keep initial goals small particularly if your child is exceptionally picky. Maybe just one or two bites of a food is enough to expect at first. Success is the key so make earning a sticker very easy at first and keep it fun. Allowing success via rewards early on will help motivate them to continue.*

- *Be consistent in your rewarding of stickers and rewards. Do this every day. Avoid using the reward chart to punish your child. Don't take away stickers for "bad" behaviours. Just remind them they don't get a sticker this time but they will have another opportunity later. Give the stickers immediately after the desired eating behaviour happens then praise, praise and praise and be specific with your praise when you give a sticker or reward so that your child knows exactly what makes you proud – "I really like how you tried that spinach. Well done!"*

- *Get your child involved in making up the chart, selecting the stickers and rewards. Develop a chart based on something your child loves or a favourite theme and make it together. Let them decorate their chart by colouring it in themselves or adding a drawing or photo of the reward they are trying to earn.*

- *Change the theme of the chart from time to time to maintain their interest and excitement. Children will be much more motivated when charts are made specifically "just for them" or by them. Make sure that their name or better still their photo is on the chart.*

- *Put the chart where your child can see it. On the fridge or a kitchen cupboard is a good choice. Draw the attention of family and friends to the chart so that they too can acknowledge the improved eating behaviour.*

- *Emphasise colour. While eating a lot of watermelon or carrot can be a good thing, children need to eat a variety of colourful fruits and veggies. The more colours they eat the more variety of nutrients. The added bonus is their chart will be more colourful and prettier!*

Avoid Less Healthy and Processed Foods

You may find it tempting to offer your child certain foods "just so they eat something" but if you are offering processed foods high in sugar, salt trans fats and additives, these may become their preferred food lessening their appetite for healthier nutrient dense ones.

Offer any liquids (juice, cordial, milk or even water) after meals rather than before or during the meal. Stop all drinks about an hour before meals, that way the drinks will not reduce their appetite for real food or dilute the enzymes required to digest the meal properly.

- Don't be tempted to let your child fill up on milk with the thought that, at least they are having something. Excessive milk will reduce their appetite for proper wholesome food and may contribute to respiratory & gastrointestinal reactivity as well as reduce iron uptake. Low iron levels contribute to poor immunity, listlessness, irritability, pickiness and poor appetite.

- While 100% fruit juice is better than artificially flavoured soft drinks, be aware that commercially prepared natural fruit juices are still very high in fructose (fruit sugar). The high caloric value of these juices will reduce your child's appetite for real food. Alternatively make juices from fresh whole fruit (plus some vegies) at home and offer these after rather than before or with meals. If at any time you do use commercially produced juices, dilute them 50% with filtered water.

- Avoid any processed or junk foods as they are usually very high in sugar, saturated trans-fats and calories and have low nutritional value. Just a small nibble of junk food could completely destroy the appetite of your picky eater!

- Aim to provide your child with a variety of fresh foods and avoid allowing them to fill up on processed snack foods or excessive amounts of the one food group. As mentioned above, make the healthy foods readily available and more convenient than any junk food or non-healthy snacks.

- Some children become addicted to certain foods. These may be the only foods that they will eat happily. These are typically dairy, bread, sugar and certain processed foods. Some food additives are addictive, affecting neurotransmitters (brain chemicals) and negatively affect eating behaviour, mood and immunity. Consider that this addiction could actually be due to food sensitivity.

- Once these addictive foods (typically gluten, casein and sugar) are removed, food choices often increase significantly. Source alternatives to high casein (dairy), gluten (wheat & other grains) and refined sugars. Try some alternative 'milks' such as almond, rice, oat or even organic soy milk instead of dairy. Rice, amaranth and quinoa are good alternatives to gluten-containing grains such as wheat.

- Never allow your child to eat "diet" foods or drink diet soft drinks as they contain artificial sweeteners such as the neurotoxin aspartame which will contribute to impulsive, irritable and hyperactive behaviour. The phosphoric acid in soft drinks or sodas will also impair bone growth and reduce bone density.

- Satisfy a sweet tooth with foods that are naturally sweet such as whole fruit instead of chocolate, candies and biscuits.

- Never use fast foods or junk foods as treats or bribes. They have no value in your child's diet and certainly give the wrong message about their value. These are not 'treats'. They contain many anti-nutrients and are detrimental to overall health and good eating habits.

Key points

✓ Remember that your child wants independence so offer choices. (Which plate would they like, where would they like to sit, do they want salad or cooked vegetables.)

✓ It's important to eat together as a family for at least one meal a day. (Dinner is probably the easiest)

✓ Make food fun! Try linking food with your child's interests. Let them help with the preparation and presentation.

✓ Introduce new foods in small portions with something else they like.

✓ Provide only healthy food and make healthy snacks and water easily accessible.

✓ What ideas have you found most helpful? Which ideas can you implement right now?

CHAPTER 4
NUTRIENT BOOSTING STRATEGIES

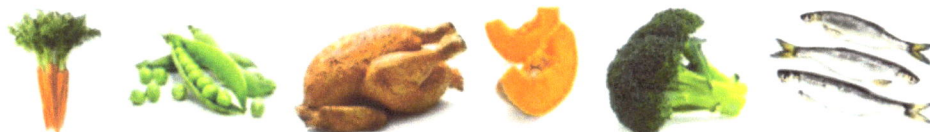

Initially it takes a bit more effort in the kitchen with food preparation when you have a picky eater but it will be well worth it. Sometimes parents need to be a bit tricky and use some strategic hiding of non-accepted or new foods into favourite foods for the sake of good nutrition.

For kids who don't eat many vegetables, sneaking veggies and other nutrients into meals can be an easy way to boost the nutrient content of little fusspot's diet.

A diet which is rich in vitamins, minerals and is provided with love is the most important gift you can give your child to be robustly healthy and happy.

Children who are lacking in or deficient in certain nutrients (and let's face it that will be a large number of poor eaters) are more likely to have eating problems or obsessions as there are certain key nutrients that directly affect appetite, food choices, and taste perception as well as mood and behaviour.

The more nutrient dense foods you are able to have your child eat, the healthier and less fussy they are likely to be. Iron, zinc, calcium, magnesium, vitamin B6, and protein are particularly important in relation to eating behaviours.

With a picky eater you often don't know from one meal to the next whether he will eat a spoonful or a bowl full so it is vital to make every small mouthful count!

Read through the list below. Maybe your picky kid is low in some of these key nutrients. If you think they may be, check through Appendix 2 for the best food sources.

Common Nutrient Deficiencies in Children

Iron deficiency is common in children and especially the picky eaters and those who drink large amounts of milk and don't have much appetite for other foods. Iron is essential for red blood cells to carry oxygen to every cell in the body. A lack of iron will show up as lethargy, poor concentration, recurrent illness and pale skin. Children require at least three serves of lean red meat a week to get enough iron.

Zinc is responsible for smell & taste perception. If zinc deficient, foods will taste bland or bad so will be perceived as very unappetising. Deficiencies also associated with recurrent infection, eating disorders and poor growth.

Calcium is required for teeth & bones and nervous system. Deficiencies are associated with eating disorders and fussiness.

Best sources are full fat dairy, nuts, seeds, tahini, leafy green vegetables and soft-boned fish such as sardines and salmon.

Vitamin B6 & magnesium stabilise mood and blood sugar & reduce irritability. B6 is required for digestive enzymes. Deficiencies are associated with mood and eating disorders.

Protein provides amino acids as the body's building blocks. Sufficient regular protein stabilises blood sugar, reduces irritability, provides energy and mood stability.

For more information on specific nutrients, their role and food sources see Appendix 2. Consult your naturopath or functional medicine doctor for more assistance if necessary.

The Game of Hide and Sneak

Sometimes you just have to be a bit sneaky in order to get extra nutrients into your picky eater's food without them knowing and making every tiny mouthful count.

To reduce mealtime battles, try some of the following

- *Use a stock or broth made from a variety of vegetables (including greens) and /or meat or chicken, as a base for a soup or casserole.*

- *Use this stock as the cooking liquid for various grains, beans, rice or pasta. At least a little of the nutrients will be passed on.*

- *Soaking grains will increase their digestibility and therefore increase nutrient availability. Try some Quinoa. Soak it first then cook in a nourishing vegetable, meat or chicken broth. It can be used like rice, cous cous or pasta. Add to any meals but is especially nice as a salad or "fried rice" with vegetables. It has a lovely nutty flavour and texture and will add a source of low reactive protein to your little one's diet.*

- *Mix finely chopped cauliflower into plain rice.*

- *Add finely grated or cooked and mashed vegetables into mince, meat balls, sausages, or pasta sauces.*

- *Bran, oats and whole grain muffins are often regarded as "cake" but are a good source of grains and fibre and are great to use as a vehicle for added fruit and vegetables.*

- *Add grated carrot, parsnip, sweet potato, zucchini or pumpkin into cakes, muffins, slices or pancakes.*

- *Adding grated beetroot makes a lovely nutritious and moist chocolate cake or slice.*

- *Pureed green and other dark vegetables such as broccoli, green beans, kale, can be disguised in chocolate cake or muffins.*

- *Pureed green and other dark vegetables such as broccoli, green beans, kale, can be disguised in chocolate cake or muffins.*

- *Top vegetables or less popular foods with a little grated cheese or a homemade sauce.*

- *Vegetables topped with cheese can be made into small homemade pizza with pita bread as an easy base*

- *Vegetable juices e.g. carrot or fresh beetroot can be added to fruit juices. These are especially yummy when made into ice blocks. Keep similar colours together for a better disguise.*

- *Puree steamed vegetables together (plus or minus some meat) until very smooth. Add to any accepted food. Only add a very small amount initially (even just ½ teaspoon to begin with) and then very gradually increase the amount each time it is presented. This method goes will with sauces, meat dishes. Bolognese or other pasta topping, over homemade pizza, into smoothies, muffins or pancakes.*

Important Note

While hiding vegetables and such in accepted foods is a helpful strategy to increase the nutrient intake of a very picky eater, it is important that you don't make these foods entirely invisible to your child or they will never learn to eat well.

Certainly use the "hide and sneak" method as insurance but, at the same time, offer small amounts of the real thing alongside.

If they see them often enough and see you eating the same thing, one day they may eat them too!

Sweeten Bitter Vegetables

If a variety of the more bitter types of vegetables (baby spinach, kale, broccoli) are offered from an early age with first foods they tend to be more accepted by children. The slight bitterness of many green vegetables actually enhances the production of and stimulates the release of digestive enzymes.

Try some of these strategies to encourage your picky eater to try them:

- *Add a little fresh lemon juice and/or honey.*
- *Add finely diced caramelised onions.*
- *Add a mix of butter, honey & cumin to carrots or any bitter vegetable.*
- *Cover with a 'sauce' made from warmed fruit juice thickened with a little cornflour, arrowroot, potato or rice flour. Fresh orange or pear juice or mango or apricot nectar are especially nice and make vegetables like broccoli much more appealing to little people.*
  Alternatively offer the sauce as a dip for dunking the vegetables.

Try some of these strategies to encourage your picky eater to try them:

- *Try making a fresh tomato sauce (blended tomatoes, a drizzle of olive oil & ½ teaspoon of sugar, honey or a small pinch of stevia) for covering less accepted foods or as a 'dip'. As the food becomes accepted the 'sauce' can be diluted a little and then less and less added to the food.*

- *Always choose fresh and young vegetables as they are less likely to be bitter and woody.*

- *Peel off skin if it is tough or is chemical tasting (e.g. apples or carrots) and remove strings from celery, snow peas and beans before serving.*

- *Where ever possible choose organic fruits and vegetables. They are pesticide free so are less likely to have a chemical taste and more likely to be in season making them sweeter and tastier.*

- *Offer raw vegetables rather than cooked. Most vegetables are sweeter when they are raw and kids usually love the crunchy texture of a raw baby carrot, green bean or baby snow peas.*

- *Dipping raw vegetables is great fun so include a healthy, nutrient dense "dip" such as hom mos, guacamole, and homemade tomato sauce or blended roasted vegetables thinned with a touch of yoghurt, olive oil or water.*

Ensure that all fruits and vegetables, raw or cooked, are washed carefully before offering them to your child. If you can't always use organic produce use a vinegar bath to remove chemical residues.

Vinegar Bath for Washing Fruit and Vegetables

1. *Fill a large bowl or basin with enough water to cover the fruits or vegetables.*

2. *Add 1-2 tablespoons of vinegar (cheap white vinegar from the supermarket is sufficient or you can use apple cider vinegar).*

3. *Let soak for 1-3 minutes then wash the produce thoroughly.*

4. *Drain and rinse in plain water.*

5. *Dry before storing.*

Favourite Textures

Children are very conscious of texture and especially in relation to food. You will notice that babies and very young children will always check out the texture of a food by hand before putting it into their mouth.

Some children like crunchy textured foods while others will prefer creamy or smooth textures. Work out your child's preference and try serving a new food in a texture that you know they already like.

Crunchy

- Try raw vegetable sticks or whole baby beans or snow peas as mentioned above and include an interesting "dip" for more fun.

- Generally children prefer the taste of crisp and crunchy vegetables so don't overcook vegetables so they become mushy. Steaming or lightly stir frying will retain more nutrient, colour and crunch than boiling or microwaving which can make vegetables rubbery and unappealing.

- If you have a dehydrator you could make your own yummy vegetable and fruit chips. Crunchy dehydrated vegetables are sometimes available at specialist or gourmet fruit and vegetable stores or delis.

- Adding something crunchy as a topping for food of less appealing texture may increase its acceptability. For example, crushed vegetable chips to mashed potato or crushed crisp breads or muesli to yoghurt.

- Some children may not like to eat crunchy foods due to the fact that sounds so loud inside their heads.

It is best to avoid using a microwave for family food. In its cooking process the microwaves alter the molecular structure of the food being cooked. This can result in a reduced availability of nutrients and over time increases the risk of nutrient deficiencies.

Crispy

- Some vegetables are more appetising when fried. That is, either dry fried in a non-stick pan or in a little coconut oil or on a tray in the oven. Instead of bought potato chips, fries or wedges try making your own with sweet potato, pumpkin, parsnip, carrot, beetroot or even beans, broccoli or cauliflower.

- Alternatively slice potato, sweet potato, parsnip, pumpkin, carrot or fresh beetroot with a potato peeler, spread on an oven tray, and spray with a little oil (optional) then bake in a slow oven until crisp. So there you have yummy veggie crisps.

- Even greens such as baby spinach leaves or Kale can be done in this way and have a lovely crispy, flaky texture while still being highly nutritious. These crispy greens are great to crumble and sprinkle over more accepted foods if your child still finds them a bit bitter.

Smooth and Creamy or Fluffy

If your little one prefers a creamy or smooth texture, present most of their food in this way, at least initially. Virtually any steamed vegetable can be mashed or pureed even broccoli, cauliflower and beans.

- Try presenting mashed or pureed foods (can have a combination of vegetables and meat, chicken or fish) as a soufflé. It will also have an egg included for extra protein and the result is a lovely light and fluffy texture that many children love.

- A hearty mixed vegetable soup also containing a little meat, chicken, beans or legumes can be pureed to appeal to a child who prefers smooth.

- Try fruit juices or smoothies with a couple of hidden vegetables. Add some yoghurt and/or some powdered protein supplement or an egg for a nice smooth, creamy consistency. These can also be frozen into icy poles or ice-cream.

Chunky

A chunky texture may be better for the child who prefers to feed themselves with 'finger food'.

- The mixed vegetable soup mentioned above left chunky might appeal particularly if interesting little pasta shapes or letters are added.

- Arrange colourful dice of cooked or suitable raw vegetables on a white plate. Try making a pattern or a funny face to get your child's interest.

- Try a combination of the pureed or finely blended vegetables and meats and form into small patties, balls or sausage shapes for the child who likes the chunkier finger foods.

Chewy

Young children and those with poor muscle tone often have trouble with very chewy foods.

- Don't overcook meats. Small children often find it difficult to eat meats which may be hard, dry and take a lot of chewing

- Offer softer meats such as slow cooked, casseroles, mince or sausages

- Make your own sausages, meat balls or patties by mixing mince or chopped meats with cooked or grated vegetables to a fine texture in a food processor. Form into the desired shapes and cook.

More Presentation Strategies

Not only the texture, but also the manner in which food is presented may make a difference as to whether your picky kid will eat. Consider and try some of the following.

Separate It

Some children prefer each type of food to be separate and not touching. I have had a number of little patients who are very specific about this. Sometimes only offering one type of food at each mini meal is the way to go. Alternatively, try using one of those divided plates or a number of small containers so that each food is separate.

Dip It or Spread It

Children love "dunking". Immersing pieces of food in a tasty nutritious dip is great fun. Dips can include hommos, guacamole, pureed roasted or steamed vegetables, pureed fruits, or yoghurt.

Spreading or smearing can also be fun for some children. Using a small safe butter knife, allow them to spread some fruit puree, yoghurt cheese or a nut butter on crackers, crisp breads, apple or pear slices.

Both methods allow little people some autonomy and independence.

Top It

Use nutritious and familiar favourites as topping for a less accepted or new food. Melted grated cheese is usually a winner. For example melted cheese over broccoli can become snow on trees. Also try yoghurt, homemade sauces, guacamole, nut butters, and pureed fruits such apple or apricot as toppings.

Wrap and Roll It

Wrap it in a lettuce, cabbage or vine leaf (san choy bow or dolmades), mountain bread, tortilla, taco, pita, flat bread, lavash, rice paper, crepes, pancakes or thin omelette.

All types of filling can be used from left over casserole, to salads, fruit and nut butter, meat and left over steamed vegetables, or an accepted filling with special nutrient dense sauce.

Your little one might like to fill it them self. Crispy tacos were always a favourite at our place. The children could make up their own combinations from the healthy alternatives provided – a savoury mince, mashed beans, grated carrot, chopped red, yellow and green capsicum, chopped celery, chopped tomato, shredded lettuce, guacamole or chopped avocado, some grated cheese and homemade tomato sauce.

Pack It

Presentation and appearance is important to young children and they enjoy the unexpected and fanciful. Be creative in how you present their food.

Try using their own tiny toy plates, brightly coloured little plastic boxes or cups.

Small noodle boxes are often a great hit when filled with little meals or snacks. These are available from the party section in many supermarkets or specialty party stores. If you can only get white ones, add some colourful stickers. These little boxes also have little handles for carrying!

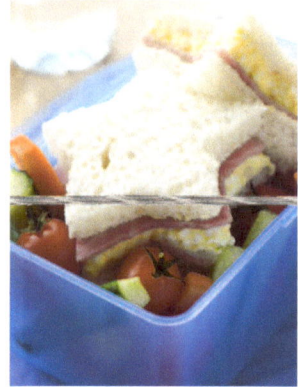

Child Size It

Present foods (especially if they are new) in tiny, pint sized portions. New foods may be accepted more readily if only very small child sized portions are served. Just a teaspoonful may be enough initially.

Make bite sized muffins, quiches and frittatas in the tiny muffin tins. For small children, use the smaller shape cutters for fish, meat or chicken shapes.

Change It

Try presenting food in different and interesting ways. Variety in presentation and texture will keep children interested and less likely to get tired of eating the same food.

Children enjoy fun and the unexpected.

For example, the same vegetable can be presented in many different ways. A plain or sweet potato can be steamed and cubed, steamed and whole (baby ones), mashed, as a soufflé, roasted, as chips or wedges, as crisps, in fingers, or cut into the shape of a star, a frog or a man.

Stab It

Food on a stick might be more appealing to your picky eater. For older children try threading chunks of fruit or pieces of vegetables on a skewer as "kebabs". For younger children cubes of fruit "stabbed" onto paddle pop stick is a safer option. Depending on your child's age, offering sturdy toothpicks or popsicle sticks to "stab" cubes of food may encourage them to try different or new foods.

Drink It - Meals in a Cup

At times children may prefer to drink rather than eat. Drinks are a wonderful way to improve a picky eaters (and your own) nutrition. All sorts of things can be disguised in a drink so don't despair!

Of course water is always the best drink throughout the day for children however you can also put a meal in a drink.

Smoothies can be made from various types of milks, juices, fruits and vegetables. They can be the basis of a really healthy meal. Nut and seed meal, protein powders, yoghurt, honey, fresh or frozen fruits and vegetables can be added and the lot blended together.

The addition of a colourful straw or drinking cup will add to the fun and compliance.

Freeze It

Most children love anything that looks remotely like ice cream, a slushy or ice block. Not all of a smoothie may be drunk at once so left over smoothie meals are easily made into icy poles or ice cream for a treat at a later time.

Freeze pieces of banana, mango, pear or other similar fruit on a paddle pop stick or in an ice block mould.

Combinations of fruits in a base of fresh fruit juice make great frozen treats. Or make up a smoothie by blending juice, milk, an egg, protein powder, fresh or frozen fruit, nut and seed meal, a little honey or rice syrup and then freezing it into "ice cream", a slushy or as an ice block.

Key points

- *Texture matters! Find out what textures your child prefers and try to have at least one of those on your child's plate. (My editor's children like crunchy so she serves raw carrot sticks and celery – great with a range of purees and dips!)*

- *Try sneaking some vegetables into meals. (A little grated carrot is yummy in meatballs and patties)*

- *Children love little packs and kits so try serving things that they have to dip, spread or wrap, or served in one of those little Chinese takeaway boxes with a special little fork. This lets them be independent and feel more in control of what they eat.*

- *Make your own fruit juice using fruit and vegetables. You can mix apples or oranges with nearly any vegetable and it will be yummy. These also freeze well to make special ice blocks for healthy snacking.*

Jot down some of the suggestions that you would like to try and that you think would work for your child.

....

....

....

....

....

....

CHAPTER 5
EXPLAINING & MARKETING FOOD

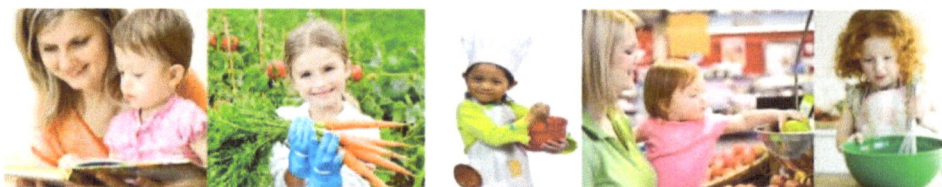

For children under three years, the best education regarding food is to continue to offer a variety of foods, be aware of their preferences of texture and favourite foods and work with those to educate their palate and ensure maximum nutritional content. Then every mouthful will count.

Later, once past three, some explanation and education regarding food and nutrition are usually needed to bring about change in your picky eater. This will give them a basis on which to progress with a more self-regulated healthy diet.

To do this, take a few clues from the marketing gurus and use some of their techniques to encourage your child to eat your healthy, lovingly prepared foods.

Even try making up some simple slogans and repeat often. Here are some that I've found.

- "Greens and beans make me strong"
- "A healthy food for a healthy mood"
- "The incredible, edible egg"
- "Apples are red, berries are blue, pears are sweet and they're all good for you"
- "Veggie juice makes me go vrrrooooom!"
- "Zucchinis terrific, like bunnies prolific"

See what others you and your child can come up with.

When talking to you child about food try to avoid using taste as an indicator of whether it is good or not. Instead, talk about how healthy it is, how it will give them energy for their favourite activity or talk about its shape, colour or texture. Try to explain the nutritional value of various foods in terms of, what's in it for them. For example, the meat balls have lots of protein or this particular vegetable, fruit or grainy bread will:

- help him grow as tall as dad
- have lovely long hair like mum
- be strong enough to kick a football a long, long way
- be able to swim very fast
- to think quickly at school and do well in exams
- bounce really high on the trampoline

Visual and Verbal Tools

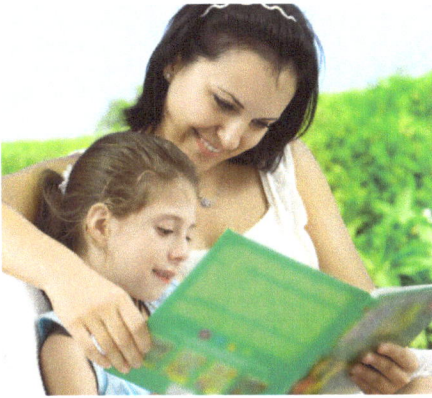

Tell your child stories about healthy eating. Read books with pictures of food and discuss this with them. Psychologists at the University of Reading in the UK found that when parents showed young children pictures of fruits and vegetables they didn't normally eat daily for 2 weeks, they were much more willing to try them when presented with unfamiliar foods.

Wander through the children's section at a book shop or ask your local librarian for help to find children's books about foods.

If you can't find an appropriate book, make one yourself with pictures and basic information cut from old magazines or from the internet.

Children watching TV will get incorrect or at best confusing nutritional information from food manufacturers advertising for certain processed foods. Such advertising is directed specifically at them. Be ready to have conversations with your child about this. My son at around 5 years had a lot of questions regarding what the TV told him was good for him, and how that differed from what I told him about those products.

Researchers, Borzedowski and Robinson, found that even a single exposure to a television commercial can influence a preschool aged child's brand preference! And Wiech found a correlation between increased television viewing and the choice of foods selected.

YOU need to be the one to inspire and influence your child so use some of these marketing tools to inspire them to listen to you more often and be less influenced by other marketing.

Explain where particular foods come from, for example the difference between fresh and processed foods. Discuss the difference between eggs from industrially raised chicken versus a free range farm chicken – compare the colour of the shell and the yolk. Explain how the bright sun and green grass produce the beautiful golden colour and increased nutrient value.

Growing It - Mini Scale Food Production

Plant a small vegetable garden in your back yard or in containers. Baby lettuce, cherry tomatoes, baby spinach, salad greens and herbs are easy to grow. Let your little one care for the plants, water them, harvest them, wash and prepare them.

Keep a couple of chickens if you have the space so your child can be involved in feeding the chickens the good vegetable scraps from the kitchen so they can make healthy, beautifully golden eggs.

This is a great way to get kids excited about their veggies and foods. A child will be more eager to eat something they have harvested themselves.

A young patient of mine recently said proudly that, "I will only eat eggs from my Henny Penny".

Her family keeps just a couple of chickens in the back yard and she loves being involved with them and collecting the eggs. While she doesn't like to eat meats she loves her eggs and so has regular health giving protein.

Field Trips

When you can, take your child on fun excursions to the source of foods. Visit small family farms, orchards, market gardens or a friend's veggie garden to experience the different animals and any crops that might be grown.

Even if a young child doesn't fully understand the concept, it may make them interested enough to try something new or retry something they have previously rejected.

Visits to local farmers markets are great if you don't have the opportunity to grow your own food or visit a farm. Here your child will see a great variety of fresh organic produce and maybe talk with the people who have grown it. Make a game of choosing a new vegetable to try at home each week. Let your child select their favourite.

Taste Testing and Science in the Kitchen

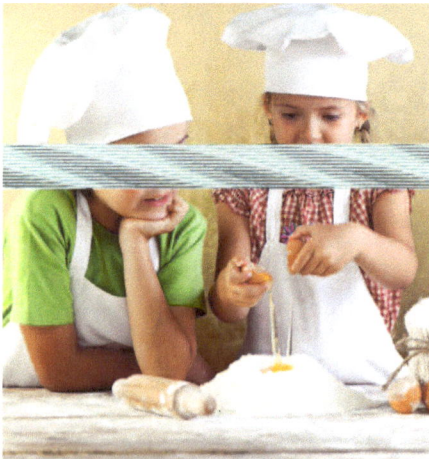

A child is more likely to eat their own creations so encourage them to take part in kitchen activities and food preparation.

Show them how to use cookie cutters to create edible designs from foods such as slices of cheese, thin slices of meat or mince patties, sheets of cooked pasta, healthy cookie dough, breads or thin slices of nutritious cake.

Add a pancake or thin cookie batter into a squeeze bottle and help them squeeze it onto the pan or a tray in fun shapes, letters, numbers or even his name.

Tell your child they are your assistant or sous chef and give them easy tasks such as stirring a mixture, washing greens, mixing the fruit salad and such.

Encourage older children to make up their own recipes. For example, smoothies with a combinations of vegetables (a little fruit added may make it more palatable initially) for the whole family.

Allow older children to watch some of the many cooking shows now so prevalent on TV. This will give them exposure to a wide range of foods, ingredients and preparation methods and hopefully stimulate curiosity for different foods and tastes. Sit with them and explain and discuss. Assist and encourage your little master chef in his or her attempts.

Key Points

- *We all know the junk food advertised to children isn't nearly as yummy as the things you could create. So think about HOW those companies are making their food so appealing. (Try serving lunch in a little box or on a plate, fork, and cup set.)*

- *Set up a little vegetable garden for them to tend and enjoy the food THEY grew. (Snowpeas, green beans and tomatoes are particular favourites.)*

- *Encourage you're child's curiosity about food. As you are cooking or preparing let them have a taste or a smell or just help out with the mixing and adding. Play games about what something might taste like, and then try it. (Taste test different kinds of apples!)*

What ideas can you implement right now?

....
....
....
....
....
....
....
....
....
....
....
....
....
....
....
....
....
....
....
....
....
....
....

CHAPTER 6
MORE SERIOUS SITUATIONS

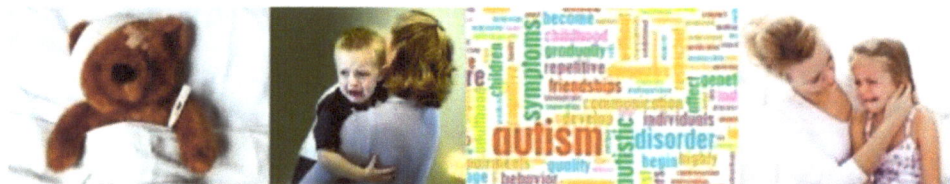

Sometimes being picky and fussy with food is more than just a developmental phase. Sometimes it may be more to do with a biochemical or physiological problem.

Food Intolerances, Sensitivities and Allergies

It's possible that your child's extreme pickiness and troublesome eating behaviours could be due to food intolerance, sensitivities or allergies. They may be reacting to some of the added ingredients in processed food or even to some naturally occurring food chemicals in fresh foods.

Food intolerance means that there is some specific reaction to a food eaten. Food intolerances are generally less severe than allergic reaction as the immune system does not become fully involved. However, intolerances can still be quite troublesome.

Food allergy, on the other hand, can be more serious as the immune system becomes involved by over reacting to a particular protein in a food and releases histamine to rid the system of a substance it identifies as a hazardous. It's the histamine that causes the symptoms of allergy.

Due to their affect in the body, some additives in processed foods are actually addictive, affecting neurotransmitters (brain chemicals) which create an increased desire for only those foods. This can negatively affect general behaviour, eating behaviour, sleep, mood, general health and immunity.

Food intolerances and sensitivities can become a problem especially if a child's diet is made up of a large amount of one particular food. Once these addictive substances are removed, food choices often increase significantly. The most common foods associated with intolerances and sensitivities include gluten containing grains such as wheat, the casein (a protein) component of dairy foods, sugar and additives in processed foods. Nuts, shellfish and eggs are also common allergens and intolerances.

Most processed and convenience foods contain artificial colours, flavouring, preservatives, saturated and trans fats as well as various other chemicals and possibly pesticides that increase the likelihood of allergic and sensitivity reactions. These may be detrimental to your own and your child's health. They tend to be 'dead' foods having little real nutritional value while further depleting your child's nutrient status just in order for his body to be able to metabolise them.

How Do I Know If My Child Has Food Allergies Or Intolerances?

The signs and symptoms of food allergy and intolerance can be very similar and may include –

- Runny nose
- Darkness and/or puffiness under the eyes
- Breathing difficulties such as snoring and wheezing
- Recurrent coughs, colds and ear infections
- Skin rash or eczema
- Hives
- Tummy aches
- Diarrhoea or alternating constipation and diarrhoea
- Nausea and vomiting
- Sleep disturbances
- Irritability and/or other behavioural difficulties
- Food addictions or other addictive behaviours

If you think that your picky eater may have some food intolerances or allergy use the Food and Symptom Diary in Appendix 3 to record your child's food intake and symptoms for 1 week. If you then find that there may be an association between food intake and behaviour or other symptoms consult your health professional for a full assessment and treatment.

Become Food Label Savvy

Learn to read food labels carefully and assess each ingredient in relation to potential reaction before you include the product in your child's diet. Learn what the additive codes stand for.

The New Additive Code Breaker, by Maurice Hanssen and Jill Marsden, is an essential tool to educate yourself and keep tabs on food additives giving an insight into the different numbers used on products to represent ingredients. This valuable little book is available at good bookshops or on line. Small pocket sized versions are also available and I have just learned that an app for food additives available for iPhones and smart phones.

You will find similar information on line at sites such as:

- *http://www.fedupwithfoodadditives*
- *http://www.foodstandards.gov.au/consumerinformation/additives/*

Be aware that nutrition claims on labels are often ambiguous or misleading and ingredients can be listed under many different names.

For example:

Sugar could be listed as brown sugar, corn syrup, dextrose, disaccharides, fructose, glucose, golden syrup, honey, fruit juice concentrate, fruit, syrup, lactose, maple syrup, molasses, monosaccharides, raw sugar, sorbitol or zylitol.

Salt might be listed as baking powder, booster, celery salt, garlic salt, sodium, meat or yeast extract, onion salt, MSG, rock salt, sea salt, sodium bicarbonate, sodium metabisulphite, sodium nitrate, nitrate or stock cubes.

Fat might be called beef fat, butter, shortening, coconut, palm oil, copha, cream, dripping, lard, mayonnaise, sour cream, vegetable oils and fats, hydrogenated oils, full cream milk powder or solids, egg or mono/di/triglycerides.

Some of these listed ingredients are well known for producing various physical and behavioural reactions in some children.

Eliminate any foods that contain artificial ingredients such as colours, flavours, MSG or artificial sweeteners.

Artificial sweeteners are neurotoxins and particularly need to be avoided. They create an enhanced response in body because they are so much sweeter and increase the craving for more sweet foods.

If the label says, 'diet', 'sugar free' or 'lite', the ingredients most likely contain an artificial sweetener and must be avoided.

Names of artificial sweeteners and their common brand names include: Sucralose (Splenda) –code955, Aspartame (Equal, NutraSweet, Spoonful, Canderel) – code 951, AcsulfameK (Sunette) – code 950, and Saccharin (Sweet N' Low) – code 954, Neotame – code 961 or simply be labelled: Contains phenylalanine.

Read the labels on everything you buy and be on the lookout for them.

You will find artificial sweeteners hiding in thousands of products including; diabetic products, crisps, cakes, biscuits, savory snacks, 'diet' fizzy drinks such as Diet Coke, Coke Zero etc, diet cordials, yoghurts, chewing gum, ready-meals, products aimed at children (low-sugar cereals etc), low-carb foods, puddings, cereals, shakes, hot chocolate, salad dressings, laxatives, gelatin deserts, breath mints and fresheners, chewing gum, toothpaste, some baby foods and even some retail vitamin supplements (chewable vitamin C for example), and children's and adult's medicine.

My general rules are:

- *The more man has had to do with getting the food to your plate, the less you should have to do with it*
- *If there are more than 2 or 3 steps in getting the food from the field to your family then don't put it on your plates.*

Remember that many of these food chemicals have an opiate-like effect in the body making them extremely addictive. If your child seems to have addictions to foods it will be helpful to consult a natural health care practitioner to assist you in assessing the problem, to find substitutes and work out a plan for withdrawing the foods.

Chronic Illness, Infection and Gastro-Oesophageal Reflux

Resistant eating may be the result of purely physical or physiological causes such as specific nutrient deficiencies, poor muscle tone, or specific developmental or congenital issues.

A large part of interest in food will be to do with smell and taste. If your child is having difficulty accepting or eating new or different types of foods they may be over or under responding to taste and smell.

Are they chronically congested? Do they have allergies? Does your child have difficulty breathing through their nose? Are they a mouth breather and do they snore? All these are likely to impact how much of their food they actually smell, feel and taste.

Another important factor to consider is whether your child may have gastro-oesophageal reflux or some other type of gastrointestinal disorder. If a child is uncomfortable or is in pain during or after eating, it is very likely they will choose not to eat. Children with very low muscle tone are also likely to have some reflux due to the weak oesophageal sphincter muscle, causing stomach contents and acid to come back up causing lots of discomfort.

Some of the signs of reflux in children include:
- *Looking or feeling uncomfortable while swallowing*
- *Frequent vomiting and /or gagging during or after eating*
- *Either eating constantly or not eating more than a few bites at a time, even if hungry*
- *Difficulty staying asleep at night*
- *Frequent sore throats, upper respiratory problems or drooling*
- *Chronic dry cough*
- *Chronic bad breath*
- *Hoarse voice*
- *Poor weight gain*

So, if your child has a known health problem such as recurrent colds, flu, ear infections, sore throats, tummy upsets, constipation, urinary tract infections, is continually irritable or has known allergies or if you suspect any of these, seek professional help.

Have all possible medical issues assessed, ruled out or treated. Consult a practitioner who has experience in treating children and has training in nutrition.

Autistic Spectrum and Selective Eating Disorder

Selective Eating Disorder is a step beyond the usually fussy eating.

The British Journal of Clinical Child Psychology and Psychiatry defines this condition as:

"The phenomenon of eating a highly limited range of foods, associated with an unwillingness to try new foods. Common in toddlers, it can persist into middle childhood and adolescence in a small number of children".

In a few people it will persist into adulthood.

With these conditions there can be an inability to eat certain foods which may be based on texture or aroma and accepted foods may be limited to certain food types or even specific brands. In some cases whole food groups will be excluded leading to developmental delays, problems with growth and weight gain as well as many other health related issues.

Sometimes selective eating comes on after a period of normal eating but it may be secondary to a history of early feeding difficulties.

Selective Eating Disorder is common in children with autistic spectrum disorders, in those with Obsessive Compulsive Disorder, and with autoimmune Coeliac Disease.

If you think your child is picky to this extent, it is important to seek professional help. A specialist in childhood nutrition, a child psychologist, an occupational therapist, speech pathologist or feeding specialist can offer treatment and advice and support for parents.

Key Points

- *Take the time to learn what those labels on packaging mean. Whenever possible choose the fresh option over processed.*

- *Learn to recognise the symptoms of food allergies and consider your family history. Are you or your partner allergic to any foods of have food sensitivities?*

- *If you are at all concerned, visit your doctor or a nutritional specialist. They can ensure that there are no other more concerning problems or allergies, and at the very least put your mind at ease that your child is growing and healthy, despite the fussiness.*

Do you have any health concerns regarding your child? Jot down any thoughts to tell your doctor?

....
....
....
....
....
....
....
....
....
....
....
....
....
....

CHAPTER 7
IS MY CHILD GETTING THE REQUIRED NUTRIENTS?

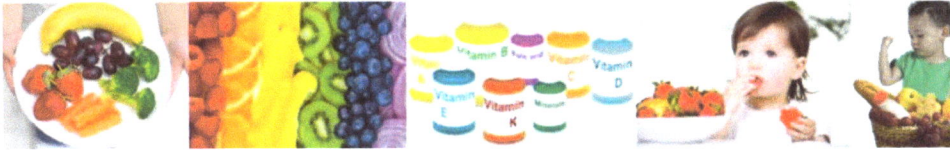

Young children tend to eat according to their own natural instincts regarding what, when and how much they need to eat. Your child's appetite will normally adjust to the amount and type of food that provides the energy and nutrients that they need to grow and thrive.

One of the best indicators of whether there is a serious health or feeding problem is their overall growth pattern. Children follow a generally expected rate of growth in terms of height and weight and any interruption to this may signal a problem. If you are concerned about your child's nutrient status check off the list below.

Your check list in assessing your child's requirement for extra nutritional support.

- *Are they growing well?*
- *Are they within the normal percentiles for height and weight for their age?*
- *Are they going through their developmental milestones as would be expected?*
- *Do they have good energy and concentration for their age?*
- *Do they sleep well?*
- *Are they generally happy and rarely irritable?*
- *Are they happy to play and share with others?*
- *Are they generally well and free from infections, tummy upsets and other health conditions?*

If you have not ticked all the boxes above or this is not the case 100% of the time for your child, they may need some further investigation and nutritional support.

A full medical and social history with a thorough dietary assessment by nutrition specialist will give some clues to their nutritional status. Blood tests will also give valuable information for nutritional assessment but are invasive and can be traumatic a young child.

See Appendix 2 for a list of nutrients, their role and foods that contain them. Use this as a guide to include more of the foods containing the nutrients your child requires. If you are still not sure, consult a practitioner with experience in childhood nutrition.

The Place for Nutritional Supplements

If your child always heartily eats a good variety of food across the main food groups and is never sick, it is likely that they need very little extra supplementation.

A good balanced diet theoretically should provide your child with not only vitamins and minerals but also fibre, fluids, phytonutrients, antioxidants and trace elements and they will absorb their nutrients best from food. However, if your child is fussy and picky regarding food and has a very restricted diet, is regularly sick or has specific health issues such as allergies or other health conditions that impact the way food is absorbed, then additional nutritional support may be needed.

It is important to note though that while nutritional supplementation may help if your child's food intake is very small or their choices very limited, nutritional supplements are used in **addition** to optimising diet and **must not be used in place of food**. Use supplement support while eating issues are dealt with and you are getting the food right.

If you are worried that your child's diet is leaving them low on nutrients and they are not able to improve the intake of nutrient dense foods, supplements may be an option. However, always consult a naturopath or trained health professional before administering any supplements.

CONCLUSION

Not every idea and trick here may work for you all the time. Every child and family is different and different tactics work for different aged children and different families. Pick out and use the ideas and tools that work for you both at the moment and then change your approach as needed as your child's eating habits change.

This can be a stressful time and it's easy to become overwhelmed:

- Don't try to do everything at once
- Set yourself one or two manageable goals
- Implement one strategy or new approach each week.

Don't panic and try to relax. In most cases your child will grow out of this phase but it's a bit like a watched kettle, the more closely and impatiently you watch it the longer it takes to boil.

Your job is to ensure the right food is available, prepare it nutritiously and serve it creatively. Leave the rest up to your child – how much, when, and if they eat is mostly up to them.

Remember some picky and fussy eating is fairly normal in toddlers and young children as they try out their independence. But there can be many other reasons why children have problematic eating behaviour. If you are concerned, investigate and rule out any health issues.

While we all worry about what our children eat, research shows that they are mostly taking in more than we think. Many children who hardly eat anything are usually found to maintain normal growth patterns are healthy and have fairly good energy. However, if you are at all concerned about your child's weight, growth or development, consult your health care practitioner.

Most children will become more adventurous in what they eat as they get older provided they continue to be offered a wide variety of foods and see that the significant adults around them eat and enjoy these foods.

Continue to be a good role model and keep as calm and consistent as possible. Make meals happy family occasions.

APPENDIX 1
The Four Major Food Groups & Requirements

Aim for your child to have some of each of the major food groups at most meals in a day. That is some protein, some complex carbohydrate, some good fats and adequate fluid (preferably filtered water).

Here is some basic information about these major food groups, also known as the macronutrients.

PROTEIN

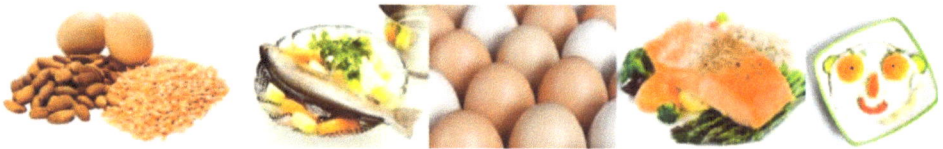

What Is Protein?

Protein is a macronutrient that can provide the body with energy. It is also used by the body as the building block for all tissue. Whenever the body has to make new tissues or repair damaged ones, protein is used as the raw material. The basic structure of protein is a chain of amino acids.

What Is Its Function?

Protein delivers the basic building blocks for the body. It provides basic structural and functional properties of all cells, tissue, muscles and organs. It is a source of energy, and is also required for the production and function of antibodies, enzymes and hormones. It also contributes to satiety, keeping little bodies full and happy, stabilizing blood sugar levels, immune system and mood.

Proteins are broken down into amino acids by digestion. Some amino acids have very specific roles to play while others form combinations to make various structural and functional elements in the body.

Amino acids are generally classified into essential and nonessential.

The essential amino acids must be obtained through the diet as the body cannot manufacture them. They do not necessarily need to be eaten at one meal, the balance over the whole day is more important.

The nonessential amino acids are made by the body from essential amino acids or in the normal breakdown of proteins.

An adequate intake of protein, containing all the essential amino acids is crucial for children's proper growth and development.

Sources of Proteins

Primary or complete proteins contain all the amino acids and are obtained from animal sources such as meats, poultry, eggs, fish, and seafood but also from a type of grain such as quinoa.

Secondary or incomplete proteins can be obtained from plant sources but do not contain the whole spectrum of amino acids. These include beans, legumes, lentils, nuts and seeds, some soy products such as tofu and tempeh. However, by combining some of these correctly, it is possible to include all the essential amino acids. For example, grains will provide a certain range of amino acids while legumes or nuts and seeds will provide a different range. By combining them, all the essential amino acids will be represented.

Try beans with rice, lentils with rice, whole grain bread with nut butter or lentils with nuts.

How Much?

Your child's protein requirements will generally depend on their age and weight. Children will need approximately 1 gram of protein for every kilogram of body weight. Protein requirements will increase as children grow and then level off as reach adulthood.

Here is an example of how a child of about 30 kilograms might get their 30gm of protein in a day

- 1 tablespoon nut butter - 2.5 gm protein
- 1 egg omelette - 6gm protein
- 1 slice grain bread – 2.5gm protein
- 50 gm cooked chicken - 15gm protein
- 1 tablespoon hummus - 1 gm protein
- 2 x 2cm cubes cheese - 3 gm protein

The main point to remember is to offer a little protein at each main meal and most snacks.

CARBOHYDRATES

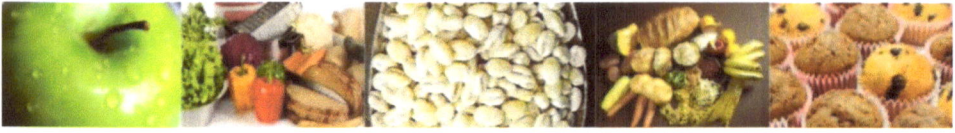

What Are They?

Carbohydrates are a natural group of substances (including sugars, starch, and cellulose) that contain carbon, hydrogen and oxygen. They provide the energy essential for children to grow, play and learn.

There are two major types – simple and complex.

Simple carbohydrates are so called as they have a simple chemical structure and the body is able to quickly convert them into usable energy.

Complex carbohydrates are so call as they have a more complicated chemical structure that results in the body taking longer to digest and use them.

What Is Their Function?

Carbohydrates are the ideal source of energy for the body. In fact, they are the only fuel that the brain and red blood cells can use and are the main source of energy for muscles. Once digested, they are readily converted into glucose, the form of sugar that's transported via the blood stream and used by the body. Insulin is then secreted from the pancreas to move the glucose from the blood into cells to be used for energy.

This process happens very quickly with simple sugars (simple carbohydrates) so one is more likely to feel hungry again very soon whereas with the complex carbohydrates, this occurs more slowly giving energy over a longer period of time.

Sources of Carbohydrates

Simple carbohydrates include the simple sugars and most refined, processed and packaged foods such as pure sugar, sweets, cakes, white breads. These foods are broken down and absorbed very quickly causing temporary a spike in sugar levels which is then closely followed by a slump, leaving your child still hungry and experiencing emotional and behavioural highs and lows. These are not a healthy choice as they usually also contain a variety of toxic additives, colouring and preservatives along with the simple sugars. Not all simple sugars are bad. Nutritious foods like fruits, vegetables and dairy products also contain some simple sugars but they also contain vitamins, minerals, fats, protein and fibre so are absorbed more slowly supporting growth and overall health.

Complex carbohydrates include the starchy whole unprocessed grains and cereals (brown rice, oats, and whole grain breads) vegetables and fruits.

The starchy and fibrous vegetables (sweet potato, white potato) are more complex. Fruits with skin such as apples and pears contain more complex carbohydrate.

These are the best choice as they allow a more gradual uptake of energy (sugars) by the body due to the more complex molecular structure plus the other beneficial nutrients including fibre that supports digestive and gastrointestinal health.

A Child's Requirements

Around 50% to 60% of a young child's food intake should consist of nutrient dense carbohydrates such as vegetables, fruits and some whole grains.

To obtain maximum nutrition, encourage your child to choose more complex carbohydrate rather than simple carbohydrate foods. Whole fruits, vegetables, legumes and whole grains (try spelt, buckwheat, amaranth, millet, quinoa, and brown rice) are most beneficial due to their nutrient density and digestibility. They stay in the body for longer, keeping little tummies full and satisfied and blood sugar more stable resulting in a brighter and happier child.

GOOD FATS

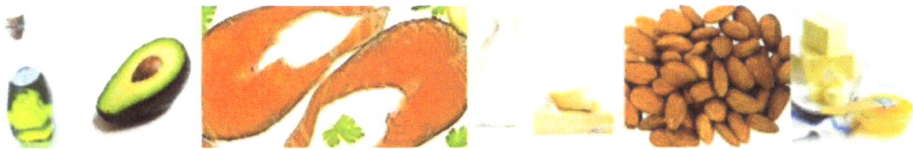

What Are They?

Contrary to popular opinion, not all fat is bad. The good dietary fats are an essential part of a well-balanced diet and crucial for your child's growth and development.

Good fats come either as **unsaturated** fats which are liquid at room temperature or **saturated fats** which tend to be solid at room temperature. Unsaturated fats include both monounsaturated and polyunsaturated fats. Monounsaturated fats are derived from plants and include olive and nut oils. Poly unsaturated fats are primarily found in vegetable oils and sea foods an comprise the essential fatty acids (Omega-3 and Omega-6) that must be sourced from diet as the body cannot make them. Saturated fats are found mostly in animal products such as full fat dairy, red meat and coconut.

The bad fats are called trans fats. They are created through a chemical process that turns a vegetable oil from liquid to solid. Trans fats have been linked to numerous health problems and have no health benefits whatsoever. They are found primarily in fried fast foods, commercially prepared baked goods (cakes, biscuits and snack foods), processed meats and dairy products, pre-packaged and certain processed foods such as margarines that contain hydrogenated vegetable oils to make the fat more stable.
These have no place in a child's diet and should be avoided.

What Is Their Function?

Good fats are essential for children's growth and development and particularly for brain and central nervous system function and to insulate nervous system tissue. Without fat, the fat soluble nutrients (vitamins A, D, E, and K) cannot be absorbed or transported.

Fat is a great fuel for little bodies. It has the advantage of carrying more energy for a smaller volume, supplying twice as much energy as protein or carbohydrates. This is why children under two require more good fat. They have tiny stomachs but extraordinary energy needs. Breast milk which is widely recognized as the perfect food contains more than 50% good saturated fat.

Fat and cholesterol are the building blocks for the structural elements of every cell and for the structure and integrity of all cell membranes in the body. The brain and other neural tissues are extremely rich in structural lipids and essential fatty acids are instrumental in the maturing central nervous system including visual development and intelligence. Considering that the brain is still developing at 5 years of age (90% developed) and a child's body continues to grow at all stages of development, good fats are a critical part of any child's diet.

Proper immune function, healing, health of the heart, lung, kidneys thyroid gland, genetic regulation, utilization of calcium for bones, and the synthesis of hormones all rely on a good supply of healthy fats.

Best Sources

Good fats are natural fats from pasture raised, grass fed animals, poultry, and wild fish. For example, quality dairy fats from grass-fed cows, such as butter, cream and whole milk, free range, grass fed chickens and wild caught oily fish. These animal fats supply true vitamin A, vitamin D and the proper cholesterol needed for brain and vision development.

Another good source are nuts and seeds and their cold pressed oils: almonds, macadamia, walnuts, pecans, Brazil nuts, sunflower seeds, pumpkin seeds, chia seeds, sesame seeds, ground flaxseeds, coconut oil and cream, olive oil, grape seed oil.

Coconut oil is extremely health promoting, supportive of the immune system and healthy gastrointestinal environment. One of its key components is lauric acid which is also found in breast milk. Coconut oil is also quite heat stable so is a good choice for cooking.

Avocado, tahini, olives along with oily fish and sea food such as wild salmon, tuna, sardines, mackerel (high in Omega-3 fatty acids) are all healthy choices.

Avoid canola and soybean oil. Unrefined corn oil, safflower oil are typically high in Omega-6 fatty acids and should only be used in very small amounts.

Child's Requirements

Current recommendations are that toddlers consume around 30% - 35% of their total energy intake from a source of good fat to ensure adequate growth and development. Lower fat intakes (<30% of energy as fat) may be associated with inadequate intakes of vitamins and minerals and increased risk of poor growth. (Nancy F Butte. American Journal of Clinical Nutrition, Vol. 72, No. 5, 1246S-1252s, November 2000).

Children from 4 years to teens require around 25% to 35% of their energy intake from good fats.

Providing a source of fat at each meal is as easy as:

- *butter or nut butter with toast at breakfast.*
- *avocado on a sandwich or as a dip.*
- *Offer fish twice weekly such as salmon, salmon cakes, tuna and other types of fish for DHA and EPA.*

If your child doesn't like fish, you may want to consider supplementation. Add a little of a particular fat or oil to soups, stews, dressings, dips or sauces

Choose foods that supply a mixture of these different fats and oils. No one fat or oil can properly suit all purposes. Children need enough of the stable saturated fats, they need enough of the monounsaturated fats or oils, and they need an adequate amount and a proper balance of the essential fatty acids, which come primarily from the omega-3 and omega-6 oils.

FLUIDS

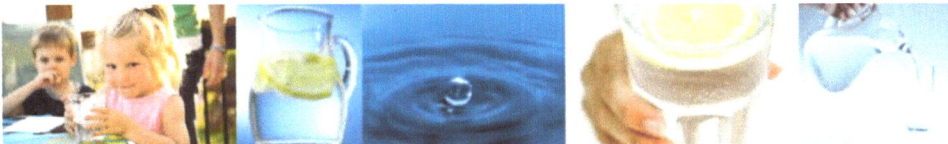

What do they Do?

Water is our most critical nutrient and needs to be your child's beverage of choice. Water is the largest single component of the body. Overall, our bodies comprise around 50 – 70 % water. Some parts, for example our brain, can be up to 85% water.

Water provides the medium in which oxygen, nutrients and waste products are transported throughout the body, through which metabolic biochemical reactions occur, through which body temperature is regulated, and how blood pressure and blood volume (85% water) is maintained. These vital functions cannot occur without adequate fluids.

Water is also a solvent, a lubricant (e.g. joints) and a protective cushion (e.g. spinal fluid). It is vital for all mucous membrane integrity preventing congestion and for proper elimination preventing constipation. Nerve and brain cells and function also require adequate water.

Even mild dehydration can cause mood alterations, headaches, irritability and poor concentration.

Requirements

Dietary fresh fruits and vegetables and vegetable juices will provide some fluids but children will need around 60ml of pure water per 1kg of body weight. This is best taken in small amounts throughout the day.

Ensure that the water you offer is as pure as possible. Invest in a good quality water filter, preferably one that is able to filter out chemicals such as chlorine and fluoride that are often added to urban water supplies.

Ways to Help Children Drink Adequate Amounts of Pure Water

- *Have a cup or bottle of water on their play table or a place that is easily accessible at all times*
- *Have bottles of water ready to take with you on outings*
- *Keep a jug of filtered water in the fridge*
- *Add slices of lemon, orange or lime and/or a few mint leaves to a jug of filtered water. This makes it more interesting and the addition of the citrus assists in hydration*
- *Freeze small pieces of fruit or mint leaves in ice blocks and add these to cups and jugs of water. Water is also a solvent, a lubricant (e.g. joints) and a protective cushion (e.g. spinal fluid). It is vital for all mucous membrane integrity preventing congestion and for proper elimination preventing constipation. Nerve and brain cells and function also require adequate water.*

APPENDIX 2
NUTRIENTS, THEIR ROLE & WHERE TO FIND THEM

MINERAL	NEEDED FOR	WHERE TO GET IT
CALCIUM The most abundant mineral. Should always be balanced with magnesium	• Bone & dental structure • Muscle growth • Nerve transmission • Hormone synthesis • Proper blood clotting • Maintenance of electrolyte balance • Regulation of cell division •	• Sesame seeds • Green leafy vegetables • Salmon & sardines (with bones) • Egg yolk • Almonds, Brazil & hazel nuts • Yoghurt & goats milk • Sea vegetables *Lost with water softeners *Depleted by high intake of phosphorus e.g. soft drinks, processed food & red meats
CHROMIUM	• Energy supply for growth • Blood sugar control • Structural & biochemical stability • Regulation of blood lipids (fats) •	• Asparagus • Egg yolk • Nuts • Prunes, raisins, molasses • Mushrooms • Oysters, lobsters *Lost in refining & processing
COPPER Problematic in deficiency or in excess	• Normal structural & biochemical development • Maintenance of skin, bone and nerve function • Oxygen transport • Regulates iron metabolism • Motor co-ordination • Fertility •	• Almonds, pecans, sunflower seeds • Whole unprocessed grains • Mushrooms • Lamb, pork, crab • Beans, prunes *Excess associated with low zinc & hypothyroidism
IODINE Problematic in deficiency or in excess	• Healthy thyroid function • Brain & cognitive function • Nervous system development • Proper immune function •	• Sea vegetables – nori, dulse Irish moss, kombu, wakame, kelp • Fish & sea foods • Iodised salt • Lima beans, mushrooms *Refined & processed foods are very low or devoid of iodine

SELENIUM	• Healthy thyroid function • Immune function • Reduces risk for autoimmune diseases and allergy • Lung development • Control of inflammation • Important antioxidant • Detoxification of chemicals • Sex hormone production	• Human breast milk • Brazil nuts, cashews • Fish, crab, oysters • Eggs • Whole unrefined grains • Alfalfa *May be low due to depleted soils and food processing method
IRON Problematic in deficiency or in excess	• Healthy vascular system • Blood health • Bone, brain & eye development • Healthy immune system • Healthy development • Synthesis of neurotransmitters (brain chemicals)	• Pine nuts, sunflower seeds, pumpkin seeds, apricots * May be displaced by excess zinc * Excess increases oxidation damage
MAGNESIUM	• Health of bones and teeth • Nerve & muscle tissue health & function • Lung tissue • Digestive process • Energy production • Calcium balance • Adrenal function • Heart function • Nervous system & mood stability	• Green vegetables • Whole grains • Nuts & seeds – almonds, walnuts cashew, hazel, Brazil, sesame, sunflower • Lima & red beans • Avocado, parsnips • Figs • Fish • Garlic * Lost through milling and processing
MANGANESE	• Bone, cartilage & skeletal development • Proper blood clotting • Development of healthy heart • Fat & carbohydrate metabolism • Intestinal enzyme function • RNA synthesis • Synthesis of thyroid hormone	• Almonds, Brazil nuts, pecans, coconut, sunflower seeds • Whole grains – rye, barley, buckwheat, corn, oats, whole wheat, millet • Brussels sprouts, olives, beans, spinach • Kelp * Lost in food processing & from use of organophosphates in non organic farming
POTASSIUM	• Muscle, nerve & heart function • Protein synthesis • Hydration • Regulation of cell permeability & pH • Blood sugar balance	• All fresh vegetables • Avocado • Bananas • Nuts & seeds • Sardines • Dates, apricots, raisins
ZINC	• Immune system development • Tissue & connective tissue integrity • Wound healing • Hormone production • Sex organ development + primary & secondary sex characteristics • Maintenance of sensory function, taste & smell perception • Proper cell division • Bone metabolism • Digestive enzyme production • RNA & DNA synthesis • Synthesis of neurotransmitters (brain chemicals)	• Pumpkin & sunflower seeds • Nuts • Whole unrefined grains • Seafood – oysters, herring, shellfish • Ginger • Meat & milk from grass fed animals * Depleted by inorganic iron supplements * Lost in milling and processing

VITAMIN	NEEDED FOR	WHERE TO GET IT
VITAMIN A In nature found as Beta-carotene Problematic in deficiency or as excess of retinoid forms	• Proper development of organs & tissues – palate, eyes, kidneys, genitalia, skin, hair, teeth & bone structure • Antioxidant • Healthy immune system • Red blood cell production • Neurological development • Steroid hormone synthesis • Regulation of gene expression • Immune function & antibody production	• Yellow & orange vegetables & fruit – carrots, sweet potato, pumpkin, capsicum, apricots, cantaloupe, mango • Leafy greens – spinach, kale • Cod liver oil • Liver, butter & egg yolks from grass fed animals • Body makes vitamin A from carotenoids in food sources * Some lost through heating green & yellow vegetables
B COMPLEX Vitamin B1 (Thiamine)	• Nervous system health & stability • Helps release energy from foods • Digestive & other enzyme production • Nerve cell function • Gastrointestinal tone • Heart muscle function • Blood sugar metabolism • Improves energy & cognition	• Whole grains & cereals • Legumes, nuts • Pork, liver • Becomes unstable with heat, roasting & light. Large % lost with milling of grains. • Depleted by diet high in simple carbohydrate
Vitamin B2 (Riboflavin)	• Breaks down fats, protein & carbohydrates • Activates vitamin B6 & folate • Growth & development • Maintenance of mucosal & eye tissues	• Maintenance of mucosal & eye tissues • Organ meats • Avocados, sprouts, broccoli, beans • Currants * Lost through pasteurising of milk & cooking of meat & vegetables
Vitamin B3 (niacin)	• Absorption of nutrients needed for growth • Energy production • Hormone synthesis • Metabolism of fats, proteins & carbohydrate • Stimulates secretion of digestive juices • Mood stabilizing	• Meat & chicken, eggs • Almonds, sunflower seeds • Salmon, sardines, mackerel • Legumes *Ethylene oxide used to ripen fruit results in 50% loss of vitamin B3
Vitamin B 5 (pantothenic acid)	• Protein metabolism • Antibody production • Steroid hormone production • Energy production • Nervous system stability • Immune function	• Avocado, beans, green vegetables, sweet potato, mushrooms • Whole grains • Egg yolk, milk, oranges * Unstable to heat. Loss in canning & freezing * Considerable loss in milling of grains
Vitamin B6 (pyridoxine)	• Metabolises protein, carbohydrate & fats • Digestive enzyme production • Brain function & mood / synthesis of neurotransmitters • Red blood cell production • Hormone synthesis • Essential fatty acid metabolism • Cofactor in synthesis of vitamin B3 • Mood stabilizer with vitamin B12, folate & protein for neurotransmitter production	• Chicken, salmon, tuna, mackerel • Egg yolk • Legumes • Walnuts, oatmeal • Whole grains * Lost in cooking & milling flour * Unstable to light

Vitamin	Functions	Sources / Notes
Vitamin B9 (folate)	• Red blood cell production & maturation • DNA synthesis & correct replication of cells - essential for production & maintenance of new cells • Energy production • Neurological development • Neurotransmitter production & mood	• Dark green leafy vegetables – spinach, kale, lettuces • Pumpkin, potato, beans, lentils • Eggs • Bananas * Loss with heat, acid, light, storage & cooking * Deficiency common with high in refined & processed foods or diet lacking diversity
Vitamin B 12 (cobalamin)	• Biosynthesis of DNA, protein & blood cells • Maintenance of bone marrow • Metabolism of fats, protein & carbohydrate • Health of brain & nerve fibres • Maintenance of growth • Mental sharpness & clarity	• Grass fed meats • Herring, salmon, sardines • Egg yolk • Requires good digestion & bacterial synthesis in the gut * Losses from heat, light, alkali & acid
Vitamin C & Bioflavonoids	• Healthy skin, gums & bones • Builds collagen, connective tissue • Robust immune system • Antihistamine • Blood cell formation • Antioxidant • Detoxifies toxins & heavy metals • Maintains cell membranes • Supports adrenal function • Regulates cholesterol metabolism • Wound healing • Protects neurotransmitter • Mood & energy stability	• Growth & mineralisation of bone & teeth • Development of a robust immune system • Protects against infection and autoimmune diseases • Cell differentiation • Proper growth & development
Vitamin D	• Growth & mineralisation of bone & teeth • Development of a robust immune system • Protects against infection and autoimmune diseases • Cell differentiation • Proper growth & development	• Proper growth & development • Fatty fish - salmon, herring, mackerel • Fish liver oils • Sprouted seeds • Whole milk, butter & eggs from grass fed animals * Is unstable to light
Vitamin E	• Normal growth & development • Supports immune function • Integrity of cell membranes • Antioxidant • Synthesis of hormones • Health of blood cells	• Wheat germ & oil • Almonds & other nuts, sunflower seeds • Grass fed beef • Egg yolk * Depleted by heat, light & milling of grains
Vitamin K	• Bone mineralisation & calcium metabolism • Proper blood clotting • Cofactor in synthesis of lung surfactant • Normal growth & development	• Synthesised in the gut by beneficial bacteria • Also found to some extent in – leafy greens – kale, \spinach, lettuces, broccoli, cabbage • Eggs, kelp, liver, pork * Is unstable to light & alkali

NUTRIENT	USED FOR	WHERE TO GET IT

Essential Fatty Acids	• Brain development & function
	• Eye development & vision
	• Development of nervous system
	• Fine tuning of all body functions
	• Proper blood clotting
	• Cell wall integrity & fluidity
	• Cognitive development
	• Blood sugar regulation
	• Regulate inflammation
	• Mood modulation (depression, aggression)
		• Omega 3:-
		    Oily cold water fish – sardines,
		    wild salmon, tuna
		    Flax seeds & oil
		
		• Omega 6:-
		    Borage/Star flower oil (GLA)
		    Evening primrose oil (GLA)
		    Black currant oil (GLA)
		    Hemp seeds/oil (GLA)
		    Nuts & seeds & oils
		    Grass fed meats
		
		* Destroyed by hydrogenation of unsaturated during processing
		* Some loss also through light & heat.

Prebiotics & Probiotics	• Stimulation & growth of beneficial gastro- intestinal microflora • Robust immune system • Good digestive function • Reduced allergy risk • Reduced risk fungal infections	• Fermented foods e.g. natural yoghurt, kefir, buttermilk, cabbage/ sauerkraut, pickles, Kombucha tea • Probiotic & prebiotic supplements * Destroyed by pasteurizing of foods

APPENDIX 3
Diet & Symptom Diary for Food Intolerance Or Allergy

CHILD'S NAME .... DATE COMMENCED ....

DAY/DATE TIME	ALL FOOD AND DRINKS (NOTE DETAILS & QUANTITIES)	SYMPTOMS, COMMENTS, SIGNIFICANT EVENTS

REFERENCES

BOOKS

Cooking to Heal - Julie Matthews
Deceptively Delicious – Jessica Seinfeld
Essentials of Nutrition and Diet Therapy – Williams
Fats That Heal Fats That Kill - Udo Erasmus
Feed Your Kids Right – Lendon Smith
Food & Nutrition – Mark Wahlquist
Healing the Hyperactive Brain - Michael Lyons
Healing With Whole Foods - Paul Pitchford
Just Take a Bite - Lori Ernsperger & Tania Stegen-Hanson
Naturally Healthy Babies and Children - Aviva Romm
Nourishing Hope - Julie Matthew
Nourishing Traditions – Sally Fallon & Mary Enig
Nutritional Influences on Illness - Mervyn Werbach
Real Food for Healthy Kids – Tanya Wenman Steel & Tracey Seaman
Secrets of Feeding a Healthy Family – Ellyn Satter
Superimmunity for Kids - Leo Galland
Textbook of Natural Medicine - Pizzorno & Murray
The Family Nutrition Book – William Sears
The Natural Way to Better Babies - Francesca Naish & Janette Roberts
The Nutrient Bible - Henry Osiecki
The Physicians Handbook of Clinical Nutrition – Henry Osiecki
The Sneaky Chef – Missy Chase Lapine

RESEARCH PAPERS

B.R. Carruth, PhD, et al, The Phenomenon of "Picky Eater": A Behavioral Marker in Eating Patterns of Toddlers - J Am Coll Nutr April 1998 vol. 17 no. 2 180-186.

B.R. Carruth, P.J. Ziegler, A. Gordon, S.I Barr, Prevalence of picky eaters among infants and toddlers and their caregivers' decisions about offering a new food. J Am Diet Assoc. 2004 Jan;104(1 Suppl 1):s57-64.

A. Wakefield, The gut-brain axis in childhood development disorders -J Paediatric Gastroenterology and Nutrition 2002 34:S14-S17.

*JE Shim, J Kim, RA Matha*i, Associations of infant feeding practices and picky eating behaviors of preschool children - Journal of the American Dietetic Association, 2011.

AJ Mascola, SW Bryson, WS Agras, Picky eating during childhood: A longitudinal study to age 11years - Eating behaviors, 2010.*C Jacobi et al* – Behavioral Validation, Precursors, and Concomitants of Picky Eating in Childhood - Journal of the American Academy of Child & Adolescent Psychiatry Volume 42, Issue 1 , Pages 76-84, January 2003.

BR Carruth, JD Skinner, Revisiting the picky eater phenomenon: neophobic behaviors of young children - Journal of the American College of Nutrition Volume 19, Issue 6, 2000.

C Jacobi, G Schmitz, WS Agras - Is picky eating an eating disorder?, International Journal of Eating Disorders Volume 41, Issue 7, pages 626–634, November 2008.

NR Reau, YD Senturia, SA Lebailly, Infant and Toddler Feeding Patterns and Problems: Normative Data and a New Direction. Journal of Developmental & Behavioral Pediatrics: June 1996.

BR Carruth, J Skinner, K Houck, J Moran III, The phenomenon of "picky eater": a behavioral marker in eating patterns of toddlers - Journal of the American College of Nutrition Volume 17, Issue 2, 1998.

USEFUL WEB SITES

http://www.parenting.com
http://www.funkylunch.com/
http://www.superhealthykids.com
http://www.littlestomaks.com/
http://domesticcharm.blogspot.com.au/
http://janette.drost.ca/recipes/
http://health.kaboose.com
http://mercola.com
http://askdrsears.com
http://raisingchildrennetwork.com
http://kidspot.com.au
http://www.fruitrhymes.com/nursery-rhymes-fruits.htm
http://theartofnutrition.com/
http://www.youtube.com/watch?v=ZD5BfC36bds, learning vegetables
http://www.youtube.com/watch?v=2IVR8BrUESQ, Lets Learn Fruits & Vegetables -
Preschool Learning

USEFUL KITCHEN TOOLS

Good quality blender

Juicer

Dehydrator

Good quality non-stick frypan

Casserole dishes & Dutch Oven

Good quality saucepan and steamers

Cookie cutters of many shapes and sizes

Different shaped ice cube moulds

Popsicle mounds

Food processor

Spirooli /Spiraliser

Mandolin for fine slicing, grating
& julienne